MUAY

WINNING STRATEGY
ULTRA FLEXIBILITY & STRENGTH

Master Lee

A catalogue record for this book is available from the British Library.

ISBN: 978-1-312-84317-2

Fifth Edition 2015.

The author does not assume any responsibility for the use or misuse of the information contained in this book.

As the primary purpose of this book is to unite all styles of Thai martial arts, the origins of each posture have not been included.

Every effort has been made to describe the postures accurately.

Information: www.MUAY.org.uk
Contact: muaymasterlee@yahoo.co.uk

Credits
Author: Lee James Crawford.
Art: Master Lee (based on photos by Angela Liu and Lee Crawford).
Editing: Angela Liu.
Testing postures: All at the MUAY organisation.
Name translations: Master Lee.

Dedication

To the readers and students:
May you find oneness and peace.

For Ange

Contents

Introduction

How to Use This Book

Warm Up and Energize Postures

Warm Up

Cat Stretch

Vitalize After Meditation

Centre Life Force

The Postures

Lower

Achieving Extraordinary Energy and Power

The Routines

Train in Harmony with Nature

Strategies

Essentials of Muay Training

Nine Lethal and Easy to Learn Muay Strikes

The Techniques

Recommended Places to Train in Thailand

Acknowledgments

First and foremost, I wish to thank Angela Liu for all her help and support. Thank you all the way.

I must also thank Tony Jaa, who after meeting at the Ong Bak film opening night in Bangkok, inspired me to start training in all styles of Thai Martial Arts.

I wish to acknowledge the support provided by Bird at the Muaythai Institute and Master Woody at the Muay Thai Conservation Centre of Thailand. Your efforts in promoting and preserving the martial arts of Thailand is greatly appreciated.

Finally, I would like to express my deep gratitude to all the masters in Thailand who have shared with me their wisdom and knowledge.

In keeping my promise to my masters, I will not write down the fatal deadly ways and will keep them secret until someone is ready and asks.

Introduction

If you have courage and commitment, this book will guide you to train your body and mind in the ways of the ancient Thai warrior, preparing you for life and the battlefield.

Muay primarily defends you against disease, illness and injury.

The exercise postures of Muay also give you movements that you can use as weapons to defend yourself.

The postures and methods help achieve longevity, energy and beauty.

Imagine gaining the flexibility and strength to have the freedom to move in any way without limitations, enabling you to do all the moves you want to do in martial arts or daily life with ease. Training in Muay can give you this ability.

This is the first time these exercise postures have been written down and include many unique and secret movements. This book has been compiled from over two thousand years of its history, the many different varieties of Muay and the thousands of training gyms/camps in Thailand.

Note- The ancient and modern ways of training in Thailand may have been influenced by nearby countries such as India and China.

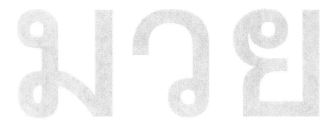

Freedom to Move

Training in Muay has no limitations on movement set by others, nor on where or when you train. In Muay, you have the freedom to move.

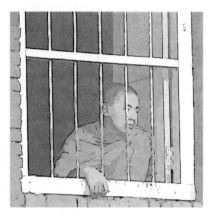

Muay allows you to train in a natural way with faith and confidence.

The freedom to move in Muay gives you strength through your whole range of motion. The muscles are trained in a natural way to become flexible, relaxed and fast to give you the power and strength you need. This type of strength gained is similar to that of the big cats and the other most powerful mammals on earth.

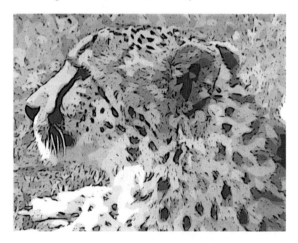

With regular training there will be no more frustrations with advance movements, tight or weak muscles. Train in Muay consistently and you will be rewarded with the gift of having the freedom to move.

About Muay

The definition of Muay is "union", to create oneness and has become commonly known to mean "boxing". The word Muay originates from an ancient language which means "pull together to form unity", for instance pulling all the strands of hair together to create a bun, which was a popular hair style in the ancient times called Muay pom.

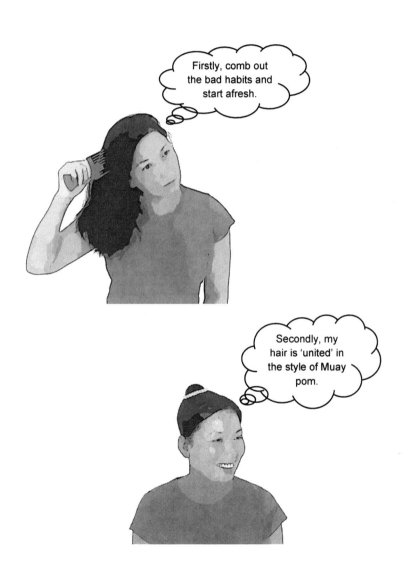

11

In Muay, the body and mind are united to give total power and create wholeness. There is an understanding that everything is interconnected. There is no isolation in Muay. You cannot break the banana plant with just your shin. The more the body and mind are united, the easier it is to break the plant.

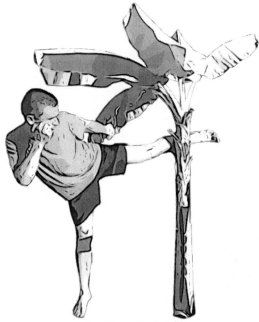

Traditional training

In Muay, the more friends you become united with, the more powerful you become.

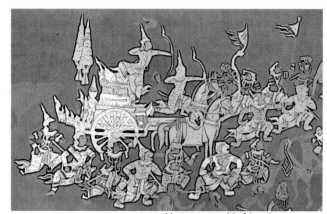

Hanuman   Hanuman with friends

The ultimate aim of Muay is finding oneness, to unite with all (connecting with everything in the universe).

Originally the martial arts of Thailand were only known as MUAY.

Each style of Thai martial arts is powerful and exciting and when they become united to form one, they become even more so.

The many styles are listed below:
Muay Boran (Ancient Muay) Many varieties including some of the following:
Muay Chaiya (regional)
Muay Lopburi (regional)
Muay Korat (regional)
Muay Pra Nakorn (regional)
Muay Chaiyuth (Winning Strategy)
Muay Luang (Royal Muay)
Muay Lerdrit (Military Muay Thai)
Muay Khotchasan (Elephant style)
Muay Kaad Chuek (Bound Fist)
Krabi Krabong (short and long weapon fighting)
Muay Thai (Thai Boxing).

When Muay became internationalized and modernized it became known as Muay Thai. It is practised all over the world and is a major influence in MMA (Mixed Martial Arts). Interestingly, as it contains 'Thai' (short for Thailand) in its name, it cannot be included in the Olympic Games.

The martial arts of Thailand contain strong elements of Thai culture, Thai Yoga, Thai Massage and Traditional Thai Dance.

All practitioners enjoy Muay for fitness training and self-defence. Muay prepares you for life and the battlefield.

MUAY organisation endeavours to preserve and practise the martial arts of Thailand in its true and pure form. Muay organisation aims to once again unite and mix all styles of old and new. MMMA (Mixed Muay Martial Arts) becomes MUAY. 100% of what is taught is either ancient or modern Muay.

How to Use This Book

Firstly, always warm up using the guide in this book or do a Muay Dance *(Ram Muay)* also known as Respect Teacher *(Wai Khru)*.

Then focus on mastering the technique of each posture followed by practising ways to achieve extraordinary energy and power.

In Muay, it is firmly believed that you must repeatedly practise a posture at least 3000 times before you can master it. This enables you to be totally proficient and instinctive. Also, it gives your opponent something to fear. Though just mastering the posture itself is not enough. You need to train daily in the ways of extraordinary energy and power to gain strength, flexibility, wisdom and so on.

Aim for refinement rather than perfection.

You may start off with loads of enthusiasm but save that enthusiasm for later when you are having a tough or lazy day.

The book suggests a few routines but you may wish to design your own to focus on what you want to achieve.

The secret to getting results is practise, practise and more practise!

Start each training session afresh and with an open mind, making it easier to learn. Treat each session like your first.

Be free from plans and expectations. Respond freshly from moment to moment.

Muay training will enable you to explore your body and mind.

Expect to learn even more when you practise. Be aware of your feelings as they will be an excellent guide for you. Feel the power when your body and mind works in union.

Ideally you should train outdoors on the bare ground. This is the traditional way but if you do not have the luxury of that as a choice or the weather conditions are unsuitable, you may wish to train indoors and use a Yoga mat, which will give you the comfort and grip that is required.

This book's content and layout are designed in the belief that simplicity is powerful and useful.

The Posture Guide

Start off by studying the pictures to give you an overall sense of the posture. The notes will then guide you through each one.

Be positive even if you are far from achieving what is illustrated. Remain positive and visualize yourself doing the perfect posture. This will help you gain faster results.

Once you start to do the postures you can begin to feel and understand the meaning of Muay, as your whole body and mind train in union. As everything starts to complement each other, you will be rewarded with lots of benefits.

All the postures have been categorised to enable quick reference and ideal usage.

Name of Posture

The Thai names have been translated into English and often describe the technique in an exciting and fun way. This will help you to remember the technique. The Thai word for posture is *Tha*. Both the Thai name and English translation are provided. The words have been transcribed using the Royal Thai General System.

Preparation: Guides you on an effective position to begin.

Movement: Instructs you on how to do each posture and technique with explanations and illustrations. Some postures consist of different parts. Aim to eventually combine each part into one flowing movement. The postures need to be firm and comfortable.

Master Lee is pictured demonstrating each posture and technique. When learning the self-defence techniques you may find it useful to visualize the other warrior as your opponent.

Technique is important. Ensure to get it right at the start to create a good habit.

Focus: This provides tips to help you be mindful of the important aspects of the movement to enhance your technique.

There are two forms to most of the postures and where applicable, these have been described.
Active Form: This form of the posture involves a flowing non-stop movement. It focuses mainly on increasing strength through the whole range.

Passive Form: This form of the posture involves maintaining the position at the edge of your range of movement. It mainly focuses on increasing flexibility by training the edge of the posture.

Guidance on how to synchronize your breath with the movements.

Inhale:
1.   Expands and opens up the front of your body.
2.   Rest and soften in posture.

Exhale:
1.   Compresses the front and side of your body.
2.   Relax to go deeper into the posture.

Channel and Intensify Life Force: Advises you on where to focus your energy and includes illustrations to help you visualize energy lines.

Purpose: This explains the purpose of the posture.

Muscular Area: Lists parts of the body where you will be aiming to gain strength and flexibility. Only areas of the body are listed. Specific muscles are not included because it depends on how deep you go, how relaxed you are in the posture and everyone is different.

Benefit: Details the benefits believed to be gained, including the internal systems and organs that become healthier and better protected.

Self-Defence: Includes some of Muay's attack and defence moves that the posture will train you for. Also guides you in how to transform some of the postures into powerful self-defence movements. It can be frustrating not having the ability to perform some of Muay's techniques including advanced ones or master tricks. Training in the Muay postures can give you that ability and freedom to move.

Interest: The postures are mainly influenced by nature and imitate movements that harmonize with the elements of nature.

It also gives interesting facts about the postures, for example, the way they mimic the movements of animals in nature or characters from the Ramakien. The Ramakien (Glory of Rama) is a historical Thai epic derived from the seven book long Indian Ramayana. The epic story is about the many adventures of King Rama and his friends.

Variation: Technique adaptions and variations for different skill levels and similar alternative movements are explained.

Take Care

Always practise Muay in a positive spirit. Practise with awareness and respect for your body's weaknesses and strengths.

Practise slowly and with control, applying utmost caution on all the postures.

The less ego you have, the less chance you are to have an injury and so the less chance you will have enemies.

The ego can be a dangerous enemy and prevents many warriors from excelling.

Stretch yourself, do not stress.

Warning- Water is an essential ingredient of ours. The body of an adult contains 60-70% water and interestingly, babies contain 70%. Therefore, if you sweat lots, drink lots.

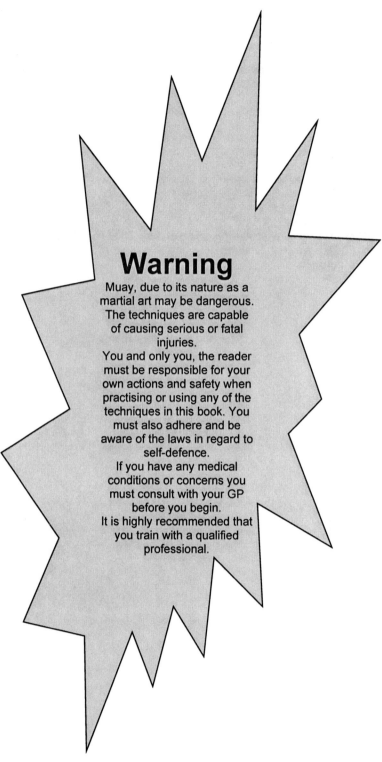

Warning

Muay, due to its nature as a martial art may be dangerous. The techniques are capable of causing serious or fatal injuries.

You and only you, the reader must be responsible for your own actions and safety when practising or using any of the techniques in this book. You must also adhere and be aware of the laws in regard to self-defence.

If you have any medical conditions or concerns you must consult with your GP before you begin.

It is highly recommended that you train with a qualified professional.

Enjoyment (Sanuk)

As well as taking care, it is also vital to have fun when training and learning from this book. You can use the Thai way of *Sanuk* to do this. *Sanuk* in Thai means having fun and enjoyment and it can be applied to other things you do, for example, work. No one wants to do something that is not fun. *Sanuk* is the art of making something that perhaps is not enjoyable into something that is pleasant, amusing, entertaining or fun.

Your spirits can be raised when practising Muay. It can give you feelings of joy and happiness. It also can make you aware of how amazing the human body is.

How- Even the toughest of training sessions can involve *Sanuk*. It can be achieved by being light hearted, having a good sense of humour and even singing.

The greatest Muay warrior is the one who is happiest.

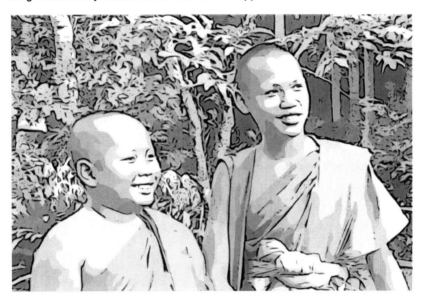

Warm Up and Energize Postures

Warm Up

These postures are to be done at the start of the routine to prepare your body. They increase the flow of vital energy and open up the main gateways of energy in the body. No matter how lazy or tired you may feel before training, be assured and remind yourself that when your vital energy starts to flow, you will feel much better.

Shortened Body Posture

ท่ากายาย่นย่อ

Tha = Posture; *Ka Ya* = Body; *Yon Yo* = Shortened

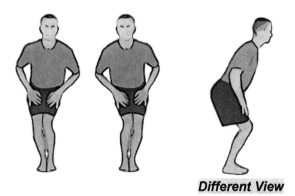

Different View

Preparation: Stand with your feet close together, knees bent and your hands placed above your knees.

Movement: Rotate your knees together round in a circle. Rotate equally in both directions.

Focus: Maintain a lengthened spine. Wide circles.

Inhale and Exhale: Natural breath movement (not synchronized with the movement).

Channel and Intensify Life Force: Energy moving round in a wide circle.

Purpose:
Muscular Area: Ankles / Knees.
Benefit: Mobilizes the gateways of life force in the knees to increase the flow of energy in the lower part of the body / Prepares the body for postures and techniques / Releases tension.
Self-Defence: Toughens knees for strikes and ankles for pivoting.

Stir the Energy Posture

ท่ากระตุ้นพลัง

Tha = Posture; ***Kratun*** = Stir; ***Phalang*** = Energy

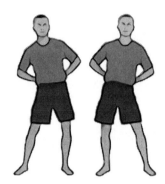

Preparation: Stand in a shoulder width stance. Knees soft.

Movement: Rotate your hips round in a circle. Rotate equally in both directions.

Focus: Wide circles.

Inhale and Exhale: Natural breath movement (not synchronized with the movement).

Channel and Intensify Life Force: Energy moving round in a wide circle.

Purpose:
Muscular Area: Hips / Core-abs and back.
Benefit: Mobilizes the gateways of life force in the hips and waist to increase the flow of energy in the core of the body / Releases tension / Prepares the body for postures and techniques.
Self-Defence: Freedom to move in your waist allows many of the Muay techniques to become more powerful / Movement of the waist can avoid attacks.

Interest: A flexible and strong core was respected and admired in ancient Thailand. This is often illustrated in Thai art with people having beautiful slim waistlines.

Charging Army Posture

ท่ากองทัพทะยาน

Tha = Posture; ***Kong Thap*** = Army; ***Thayan*** = Charging

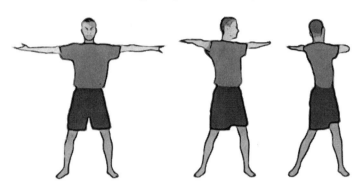

Preparation: Stand in a shoulder width stance and raise your arms out to the sides so that they are level with your shoulders.

Movement: Swing your body from side to side. To advance the posture on each swing your lead palm needs to be facing down and the following palm facing up.

Focus: Maintain softness. Tune into how your energy feels.

Inhale: As you return.   *Exhale:* As you twist round.

Channel and Intensify Life Force: Energy moving round, radiating from your core, through your finger tips and beyond.

Purpose:
Muscular Area: Back / Shoulders / Neck.
Benefit: Mobilizes the gateways of life force in the torso to increase the flow of energy in the upper part of the body / Invigorates spine / Prepares the body for postures and techniques / Flow of energy to your head / Increases energy / Nervous system / Eye focus / Releases tension.
Self-Defence: See p.168 for details on how to use this movement in battle.

Variation: Pivot on the ball of the foot to increase movement. You can also practise this posture with your head always facing forward.

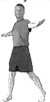

Deer Looks Back Posture

ท่ากวางเหลียวหลัง

Tha = Posture; *Kwang* = Deer; *Liao* = Turn the head to look; *Lang* = Behind

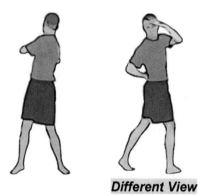

Different View

Preparation: Stand in a shoulder width stance.

Movement: Twist your body round to look behind. Place one hand on your lower back and your other hand above your eyes as if to shade the light. Repeat on the other side.

Focus: Widen your awareness as you look. Close your eyelids very slightly and see the whole area around you.

Inhale: To return.

Exhale: As you twist round.

Channel and Intensify Life Force: Energy moving round, radiating from your core.

Purpose:
Muscular Area: Back / Shoulders / Neck.
Benefit: Mobilizes the gateways of life force in the torso to increase the flow of energy in the upper part of the body / Invigorates the spine / Prepares the body for postures and techniques / Flow of energy to head / Increases energy / Nervous system / Eye focus / Releases tension.
Self-Defence: Prepare for spinning techniques / Master tricks / Eye focus in battle.

If you are in a situation where you miss an attack, for example a kick, or have your back turned to your opponent, you can apply the master trick called Deer Looks Back. Simply turn back and use a side push kick.

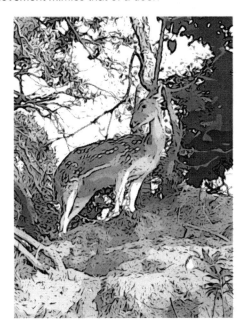

The posture also emulates another variation to the master trick. When your back is turned from your opponent, simply do the same as the posture. Whilst you look back with one of your forearms shielding your head, your other elbow rises up to attack with a reverse elbow strike targeting your opponent's chin.

Interest: The movement mimics that of a deer.

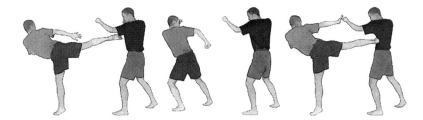

Interest: It is useful to train the focus of the eyes. With a soft gaze (close the eyelids very slightly), spread your vision to expand your awareness to what is around you. Avoid focusing on one thing. This will enable you to see more and enhance your defence and attack. It also has the effect of unsettling your opponent as you will appear more confident and focused.

Elephant Destroying the Holding Pen

ท่าช้างทำลายโรง

Tha = Posture; *Chang* = Elephant; *Thamlai* = Destroy;
Rong = Building (Holding Pen)

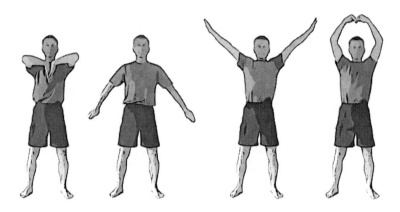

Preparation: Stand in a shoulder width stance with the backs of your hands together in downward *wai*. For details about the *wai* see p.64 and p.150.

Movement: Rotate both your arms forwards and as you raise your arms turn your palms.

Focus: Keep your shoulders down, be aware of tension arising.

Active Form: Continuous arm circles.

Inhale: As you raise your arms.

Exhale: As you lower arms.

Channel and Intensify Life Force: Energy moves round in a circle and out through your fingertips.

Purpose:
Muscular Area: Upper / Back / Shoulders.
Benefit: Mobilizes the gateways of life force in the shoulders to increase the flow of energy in the upper part of the body / Prepares the body for other postures and techniques / Upright posture / Releases tension.

Self-Defence: Defensive blocks / Swipes, blocks, opens and covers / The movement forms a double lower outer brush. When applied with speed it is an excellent defence if your opponent tries to grab you either high or low with both hands. You can follow with an elbow strike / Overhead punches / Elbows.

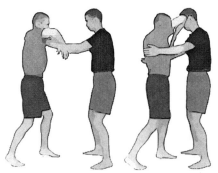

There is a master trick of the same name that is used to defend yourself in a grapple. It uses the same arm movement along with a quick bend to the side. This has the effect of off-balancing your opponent and opening up the side of their body, giving you freedom and a big target to stamp down on.

Interest: As you lower the arms, the hands form the shape of an elephant's tusks. The nature of the elephant is to have the freedom to move and this movement mimics an elephant setting itself free from a building that is restraining it.

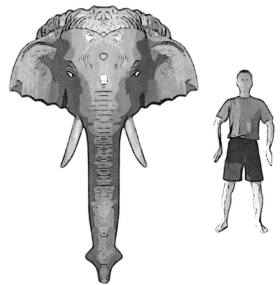

Variation: Raise your heels as you raise your arms and lower them when you lower your arms (optional).

Tiger Destroying the Hunter's Tree Hide

ท่าเสือทำลายห้าง

Tha = Posture; *Suea* = Tiger; *Thamlai* = Destroy; *Hang* = Hunter's Tree Hide

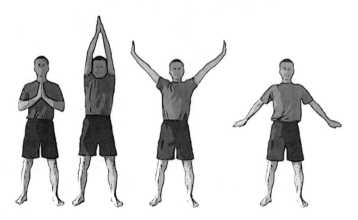

Preparation: Stand in a shoulder width stance with your hands in a *wai* position.

Movement: Rotate both your arms backwards and as you raise your arms turn your palms.

Focus: Keep your shoulders down.

Active Form: Continuous arm circles.

Inhale: As you raise your arms.

Exhale: As you lower arms.

Channel and Intensify Life Force: Energy moving round in a circle and out through your fingertips.

Purpose:
Muscular Area: Upper back / Shoulders.
Benefit: Mobilizes the gateways of life force in the shoulders to increase the flow of energy in the upper part of the body / Prepares the body for other postures and techniques / Posture / Releases tension.

Self-Defence: Defensive blocks / Swipes, blocks, opens and covers / Uppercut punches / The movement forms a double upper outer brush. When applied with speed it is an excellent defence if your opponent tries to grab you either high or low with both hands.

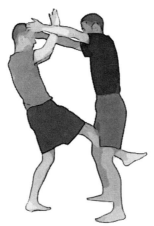

There is a master trick with the same name which emulates some of this movement. It has three parts to it and each part allows you to practise a different way of using the movement:
1st To defend against a round kick, swing both of your arms up into a *wai* position so that you shield with your elbows. The higher the kick the higher you raise the *wai*. This is the same movement that is used when holding Thai pads for practising round kicks.
2nd To defend against a swing punch, swing both your arms up so that one arm forms an upper outer brush to deflect the punch outwards, whilst your other hand pushes your opponent's mid chest.
3rd Once your opponent is off-balanced and they have a bend in their knee, you have the opportunity to swing your arms up to help you step up on to their thigh and jump high. As you drop down, strike downwards with you inner wrist, targeting their head. You can also do it by just flying upwards, taking two or three steps run up and ensuring to swing your arms up to gain height.

Another master trick with the same name involves leaning back to avoid a round kick. When the opponent's back is turned having missed the kick, you counter attack with a downwards axe kick targeting the back of their neck or head.

Both master tricks aim for high targets to avenge the shot of a round kick.

Interest: Elephant Destroying Holding Pen and Tiger Destroying Hunter's Tree Hide are Thai proverbs which refer to a discourteous person. They most likely comes from the process of hunting and taming wild animals. The animal will naturally become enraged leading to a struggle, fighting to survive and be free. The movements both originate from Thai sword fighting.

Variation: Raise your heels as you raise your arms and lower them when you lower your arms (optional).

Cat Stretch

Whenever you get the urge to stretch or become aware of tension in your body, have a quick stretch in the same way cats do. Do not let your ego limit you. Have the freedom to move like a cat.

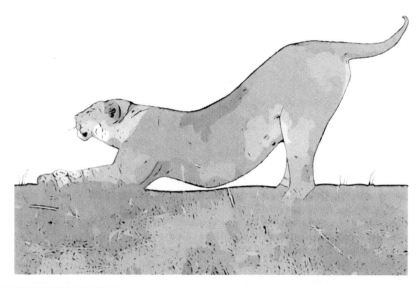

Integration Practice- The two postures that follow are good examples of quick cat stretches that you may use throughout the day. They are great for releasing tension in the back, keeping the spine healthy and supple and so believed to be vital for longevity.

Quick cat stretches are also used to prepare for training in the techniques of Muay or before a fight. They can include any of the stretches in the book and are just held for a short while.

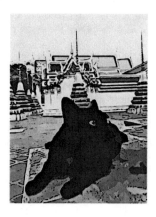

Arching Twisting and Bending Flow Posture

ท่าโค้งบิดเอียงและไหล

Tha = Posture; ***Khong*** = Arching; ***Bit*** = Twist; ***lang*** = Bending;
Lae = and; ***Lai*** = Flow

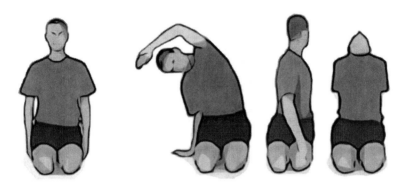

Preparation: Kneel with your knees and feet close together.

Movement: There are three parts to this posture. Firstly, bend from side to side. Secondly, twist round in each direction. Thirdly, arch backwards.

Focus: Aim to feel the stretch in all three ranges of movement in the spine.

Active Form: Continuous.

Passive Form: Train each individual part of the posture.

Inhale: Upon return.

Exhale: Bend / Twist / Arch.

Channel and Intensify Life Force: Radiating from your core.

Purpose:
Muscular Area: Spine.
Benefit: Rejuvenate / Revitalize / Re-energize and release tension particularly in the spine / Also has same benefits as side bends, twists and back bends.
Self-Defence: Agility in attack and defence.

Interest: Ideal to do throughout the day to refresh and release tension.

Variation: Another option is to do this posture standing.

Ward off Illness Posture
(Tense, Shake, Breathe)

ท่าขจัดโรคภัย ตึง สั่น ลม

Tha = Posture; *Khachat* = Ward off; *Rok Phai* = Illness; *Tueng* = Tense;
San = Shake; *Lom* = Breath

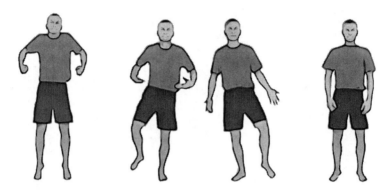

Preparation: Standing, sitting or lying.

Movement: There are three parts to this posture. Tense all the muscles in your body, then shake your body followed by a full natural breath.

Focus: You must first become aware of tension before you can let it go. Tensing up first helps you with this.

Inhale: Tense.

Exhale: Shake.

Channel and Intensify Life Force: Letting go of negative energy.

Purpose:
Muscular Area: Whole body.
Benefit: Shakes off all illnesses / Awareness and release of tension / Nervous system / Internal organs.
Self-Defence: Softness and speed in all Muay techniques.

Interest: As soon as you feel tension in the body, you may use this posture as a remedy. You can apply it before or after a stressful situation. It may also help you before you practise other postures or techniques to combat unnecessary tension.

Variation: You can tense and release individual parts of the body rather than your whole body.

Vitalize After Meditation

Re-awake and vitalize the body after long periods of stillness. These postures can also be used as part of a warm up.

Meditation Posture

ท่านั่งสมาธิ

Tha = Posture; *Nang Samathi* = To Sit and Meditate

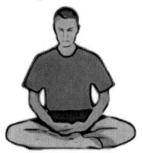

Preparation: Sit on a meditation cushion, Thai pad or block with legs crossed. Place your palms upwards, with right over left. Excellent posture is essential to encourage the natural curve of your lower back. Chin is slightly down.

Movement: The only movement is that of your full natural breaths.

Focus: Your body should be free from tension. A good posture allows the life force to spiral upwards from the base of spine.

Channel and Intensify Life Force: Forms a powerful triangular base and upright posture that allows your energy to flow well, whilst also harnessing the energy around you.

Purpose:
Muscular Area: Ankles / Knees / Hips / Spine.
Benefit: Centre energy / Mindfulness / Calming / Relax / Refresh / Restore.
Self-Defence: Mindfulness to avoid battle / Mindfulness in battle / Mindfulness to recover after battle.

Interest: See p.120 on how to train mindfulness with meditation.

Variation: If comfortable you can sit in the full lotus posture.

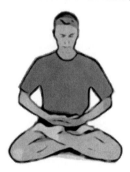

Power Summoning Posture

ท่าเรียกพลัง

Tha = Posture; *Riak* = Summoning; *Phalang* = Power

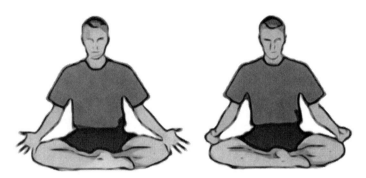

Preparation: Sit in the meditation posture. Place hands on your knees with your palms facing upwards.

Movement: Open and relax your hands followed by closing and tensing your fists. Repeat.

Focus: Release and tense the fists only and be aware of unnecessary tension elsewhere.

Inhale: As you create fists.

Exhale: As you soften and release the fists.

Channel and Intensify Life Force: Making a fist strengthens the flow of life force. Draw energy in as you make fists.

Purpose:
Muscular Area: Hands.
Benefit: Connection with breath / Increase energy.
Self-Defence: This can be basic preparation for making a fist. It is also an advanced practice of only tensing when necessary, for example, when delivering a punch you only need to tense the fist upon impact, giving you more speed and power.

Variation: If comfortable you can sit in the full lotus posture.

Mountain Peak
Counterbalance Posture

ท่าคานยอดเขา

Tha = Posture; *Khan* = Counterbalance; *Yot Khao* = Mountain Peak

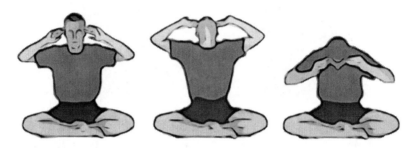

Preparation: Sit in the meditation posture. Place your fingertips behind your ears.

Movement: Arch back and at the same time draw your elbows back and look upwards. Release and bring head down.

Focus: Maintain softness especially in your legs.

Inhale: Arch and draw elbows backwards.

Exhale: Return and release.

Channel and Intensify Life Force: From the centre of your body and downwards, you must remain soft so that your energy sinks down to create a firm base, enabling you to draw energy from the earth. From the centre of your body and upwards, your energy travels up through your head and elbows and into the air.

Purpose:
Muscular Area: Spine / Back.
Benefit: Release tension in back / Revitalize / Energize / Eye focus / Focuses mind / Encourages the full natural breath.
Self-Defence: Release tension and increase speed.

Interest: The greater the mountain peak, the greater the foundations must be.

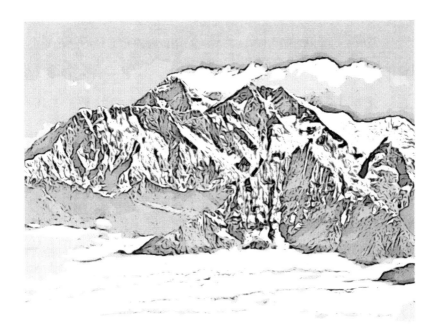

Variation: If comfortable you can sit in the full lotus posture. You can also open your eyes as you inhale and look up and close your eyes as you exhale and lower.

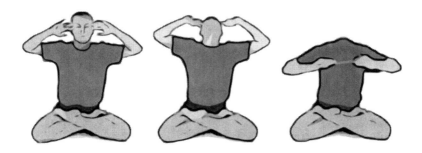

Mountain Moving Posture

ท่าเคลื่อนขุนเขา

Tha = Posture; *Khluean* = Moving; *Khun Khao* = Mountain

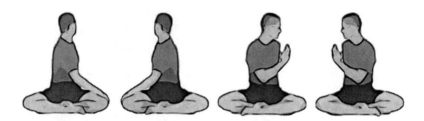

Preparation: Sit in meditation or full lotus posture.

Movement: There are two parts to this movement. Firstly, place one hand on your knee with your other hand behind. Twist round in both directions using your arms to assist. Secondly, raise your arm high and drop it down to form a single *wai*, then twist your body round to the opposite side. Repeat on the other side. Return and repeat.

Focus: Maintain softness and a good posture.

Active Form: Continuous.

Passive Form: Train the edges in both parts.

Inhale: When returning.

Exhale: When twisting.

Channel and Intensify Life Force: Radiating from your core.

Purpose:
Muscular Area: Shoulders / Back / Neck.
Benefit: Posture / Agility in back / Spinal nerves / Flow of life force to spine / Internal organs / Digestion / Refresh.
Self-Defence: Turning the core for extra power on defence or attacking techniques.

38

Centre Life Force

This is the way to centre your energy after periods of stillness or action. It can also form a flowing journey from posture to posture. Always apply the essentials of Muay even between postures. See p.155 for the Essentials of Muay Training.

Centre the Energy Posture

ท่ารวมศูนย์พลัง

Tha = Posture; *Ruam Sun* = Centre; *Phalang* = Energy

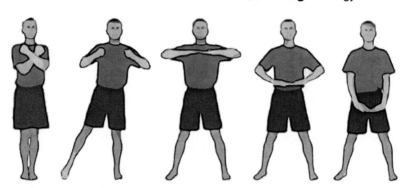

Preparation: Arms crossed in what is called a Thousand Fists.

Movement: Step and move your fists across to open the guard, then press your palms downwards.

Focus: Tune into how life force feels. Use softness to ground you to the earth. Breathe, relax, here and now.

Inhale: As you open the guard.

Exhale: As you press the palms downwards.

Channel and Intensify Life Force: Movement of energy is synchronized with the movement.

Purpose:
Benefit: Centres your energy before and after a posture or technique / Channel and control energy / Awareness / Being present.
Self-Defence: Forms one of the many protective guards of Muay ideal for deflecting attacks / Moves your feet into an ideal position.

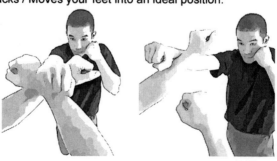

Interest: A Thousand Fists is a superb guard because from it, a thousand movements can flow effortlessly.

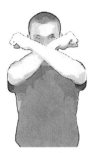

Variation: This variation illustrates coming out of a stance or posture. It is a similar movement but instead, you bring your feet inwards. It can be used with a wide or shoulder width stance.

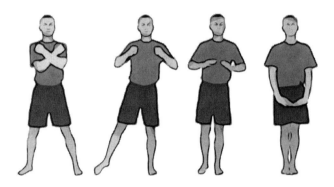

The Postures

Lower

Dance Posture

ท่ารำ

Tha = Posture; *Ram* = Dance

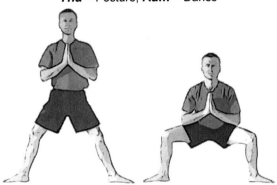

Preparation: Stand in a wide stance with your feet and knees facing outwards with a very slight bend in the knees. Hands in a *wai* position. For details about the *wai* see p.64 and p.150.

Movement: Bend both your knees. Your knees and feet need to remain in line with each other as they face outwards to the side throughout the movement. Go as low as you can and then return to the preparation position.

Focus: Keep your back upright as you lower straight down. Avoid leaning forwards. You may find it helpful to gently ease your hips forward.

Active Form: Continuous movement up and down.

Passive Form: Train on the low.

Inhale: As you lower.

Exhale: As you rise / Go deeper into the posture.

Channel and Intensify Life Force: Softness will allow your energy to sink to the earth. Visualizing energy through your knees will help keep them open.

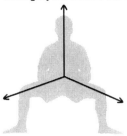

Purpose:

Muscular Area: Legs / Buttocks.

Benefit: Angular movement power in hips and legs / Opens out pelvic area / Increases longevity / Improves metabolic rate / Bone density.

Self-Defence: Strengthens stance and footwork / Knee blocks / Knee strikes / Kicks / Ducking.

Interest: This posture is also used in Thai dance and in the Thai Hermit's style of Yoga called Remedy for Longevity.

Variation: You may use a pole to assist your balance.

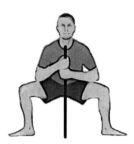

Variation: You may also practise this posture with a partner. It is called Pressing the Angles. Stay in the low position and as you exhale, your partner gently pushes their feet forwards against your knees. Be sure to communicate well.

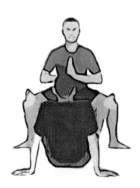

Hermit Sits on a Pedestal Posture

ท่าฤาษีนั่งแท่น

Tha = Posture; *Ruesi* = Hermit; *Nang* = Sit; *Thaen* = Pedestal

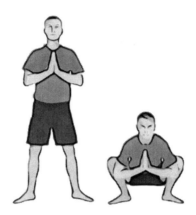

Preparation: Stand in a shoulder width stance with feet out at 45 degrees.

Movement: Lower by bending your knees. Keep your knees in line with your toes. Then come up.

Focus: Maintain good posture.

Active Form: Continuously up and down.

Passive Form: Stay low and aim to go lower.

Inhale: As you lower.

Exhale: As you rise / Go deeper into the posture.

Channel and Intensify Life Force: Softness will allow your energy to sink to the earth.

Muscular Area: Ankles / Legs / Buttocks / Hips / Lower back.
Benefit: Opens out pelvic area / Circulation.
Self-Defence: Defensive leg movements / Kicks and knees / Forms a master trick with the same name. The purpose of the trick is to defend against a round kick by sitting on your opponent's attacking leg, breaking their knee joint.

Interest: A major style of Yoga in Thailand is called The Hermit's Body Twist, Rusie Dotton, which includes 127 hermit postures. Another form is commonly nicknamed Lazy Yoga, referring to Thai Massage where a person remains effortless whilst a trained practitioner moves them through yogic type postures.

A hermit was a wise person renowned for their wisdom. With their knowledge of medicine, hermits helped many people.

The posture is also known as the Garland Posture.

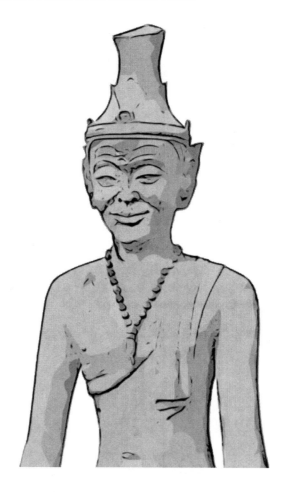

Mighty Bird Posture

ท่าพญาครุฑ

Tha = Posture; *Phaya Khrut* = Mighty Bird *(Garuda)*

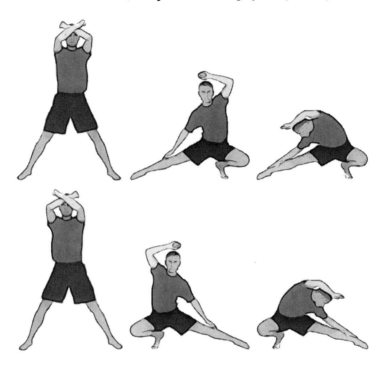

Preparation: Stand in a wide stance. Raise and cross your arms in what is called a Thousand Fists.

Movement: Bend one knee to lower. At the same time spread your arms to the opposite side. Keep your foot pointed on the extended leg. Continue the movement by rising back up. Change your guard and repeat on the other side. If you lower to the left side you need to use a left guard with your left fist behind the right. Remember to change the guard as you change sides.

Focus: Keep your knee out to the side.

Active Form: Alternate from side to side.

Passive Form: Deepen on the low.

Inhale: Raise and pull your guard back.

Exhale: Lower and spread your arms over.

47

Channel and Intensify Life Force: Through your arms and beyond. Through your knee and foot and beyond.

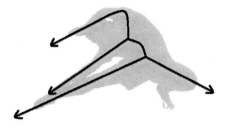

Purpose:
Muscular Area: Legs / Backside / Hips / Core / Shoulders.

Benefit: Opens up side of body / Opens up hips / Opens chest / Balance / Confidence / Awareness of boundless reserves of life force / Focus.

Self-Defence: Guard / Round kicks / Round knees / Thousand Fist guard / This will help the technique called Sweep the Earth become more powerful (see p.164).

Interest: Garuda, the king of the birds has an almighty wing span of many kilometres. Garuda's flapping wings are so powerful they can move seas to find Nagas (dragon-like serpent snakes).

In this posture your arm represents Garuda's wings reaching far and beyond.

Garuda is a state symbol of Thailand.

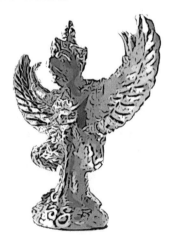

Variation: Bend over and reach in a pulse like action three times.

Salute Star Posture

ท่าชมดารา

Tha = Posture; *Chom* = Salute; *Dara* = Star

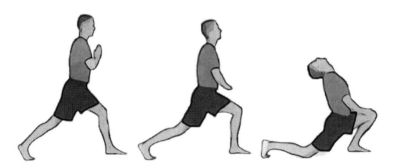

Preparation: Step into a wide stance then turn your body so that your feet are in line with the hips. Hands in a *wai* position. For details about the *wai* see p.64 and p.150

Movement: Bend your lead knee to lower, keeping the sole of your lead foot on the ground. Lengthen your back leg and foot. As you lower, place your hands on your knee. Continue the movement by arching backwards. Rise back up with hands in a *wai*. Turn your feet in the opposite direction and repeat on the other side.

Focus: Keep your hips facing forwards.

Active Form: Continuous movement, alternating from side to side.

Passive Form: Train on the low.

Inhale: Lower and arch back.

Exhale: Rise up / Go deeper into the posture.

Channel and Intensify Life Force: An arch of energy going through the top of your head and your foot. Energy also travels forwards from the hip of your rear leg.

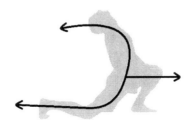

Muscular Area: Legs / Buttocks / Hips / Spine.

Benefit: Opens hip and groin / Opens chest / Eye focus with soft gaze / Balance.

Self-Defence: Push kicks / Straight kicks / Straight knees / Knee blocks / Also helps develop power in thrusting of the hips in push kicks and straight knees / Helps with a technique called Tiger Pulls Tail / *Wai* guard.

Interest: On a clear night this is a beautiful way to connect with the energy around you as you gaze up at the stars.

Mountain Embracing Posture

ท่าโอบห่อขุนเขา

Tha = Posture; *Op Ho* = Embracing; *Khun Khao* = Mountain

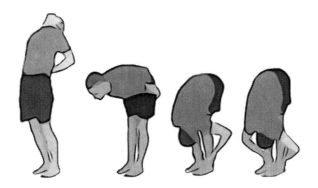

Preparation: Stand with feet close together and hands resting on your lower back.

Movement: Arch your spine back and continue the movement by folding forwards at the hips. Bring your chest to knees and head to shins. Embrace on the low and then return to the preparation position. Repeat.

Focus: Lengthen your spine. Your sitting bones represent the peak of the mountain and should be raised high up to the sky. Keep your neck soft.

Active Form: Continuous.

Passive Form: Train the edge, maintain embrace.

Inhale: Rise up and arch back.

Exhale: Fold forwards / Lift sitting bones and deepen embrace.

Channel and Intensify Life Force: Focus on the energy traveling through the peak of your sitting bones and the top your head.

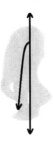

51

Muscular Area: Back of body including back of legs.
Benefit: Flow of blood to brain / Squeezing on the embrace increases the flow of life force to your abdominal organs / Calming / Relieves exhaustion.
Self-Defence: Freedom to move in kicks and knees at different heights.

Interest: For many people the lack of flexibility in the back of the legs (hamstring muscles) prevents them from being able to perform higher kicks or knee strikes. There are many postures in Muay which help you to improve flexibility in the hamstrings, enabling you to reach a higher level. If you choose to focus on this weakness it is important to balance forward bends with backbends.

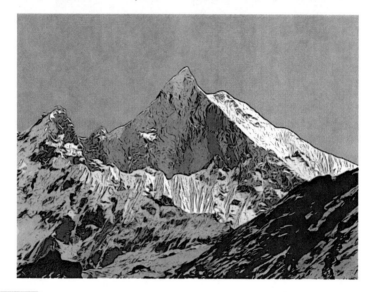

Variation: An excellent way to prepare for this posture is to embrace your legs with your knees bent before you extend the legs. This allows you to get the full benefits and feeling of the embrace. Your hands can be in a *wai* position or you can grab your ankles.

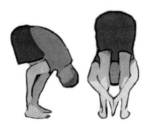

Monkey Crosses Over to Lanka Posture

ท่าหนุมานข้ามลงกา

Tha = Posture; *Hanuman* = Great White Monkey; *Kham* = Crosses Over; *Longka* = Lanka

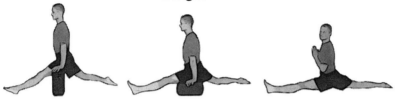

Preparation: Kneel on the ground, step one leg forward and the other leg behind. Depending on your flexibility, put your hands on the ground or on to a stable object for example, a Thai pad. Use your hands to support your bodyweight. You may find it helpful to prepare your body first by doing the passive forms of the Mountain Embracing and Salute Stars postures.

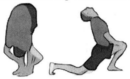

Movement: Lower to the ground. Raise the hands in a *wai* position when you are able to relax your legs on the ground.

Focus: Maintain good posture with the natural curves of the spine. Your feet, knees and hips all need to be in alignment.

Active Form: When you are comfortable at the edge of the movement, push the heel of your lead foot down into the ground and at the same time, push the front of the foot down on the back leg. This will increase strength in that specific range of movement.

Passive Form: Relax at the edge to take the legs further apart.

Inhale: Prepare / Rest / Return.   **Exhale:** Sink and release into posture.

Channel and Intensify Life Force: Focus on spreading both legs wide in opposite directions and allow your energy to sink down.

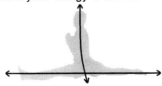

53

Purpose:
Muscular Area: Back of legs / Front of hips.

Benefit: Balance in the lower body / Circulation in legs / Overcome fear / Opening your legs and hips wide opens your mind up to possibilities / Awareness of imbalances / Opens up chest.

Self-Defence: Once you can do the splits it opens up the possibility of doing the advanced techniques that require a wide freedom of movement / High kicks / High knees / There is a master trick with the same name, which requires great agility (like that of a monkey) to step over a low round kick and jump towards the opponent with a flying knee. It forms the method of doing a jumping knee by lifting your opposite knee up first to help you launch forwards and upwards. The technique is also hidden in Thai dance drama. It can also be seen in a variation which involves stepping completely over the enemy by first stepping up onto their upper leg and then their shoulder, giving a high stunt like flying knee aimed at another opponent.

Interest: The great white monkey is Hanuman who is one of King Rama's most loyal soldiers.

The movement resembles a scene from the Ramakien where Hanuman travels to Lanka to return a magic ring back to Sida (wife of King Rama). The journey becomes a challenge when he reaches a wide waterway that seems impossible to cross. Hanuman uses the powers of courage and faith to gain size and stretch his tail across the waterway to form a bridge. This amazing feat allows his monkey army to unite with him. His guide for the journey is a hermit.

When training to do the splits, one must always have courage and faith like Hanuman. It is possible that you can do the splits. You must believe. We all have the ability. We all have the hip structure that will allow us to do it. So unless you have a permanent injury, illness or disease, you can achieve the splits. With practise you can do it!

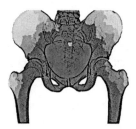

Variation: If you are less flexible in the back of the legs you may wish to focus more on that area by leaning forwards. To focus more on the flexibility of the front of the hip, lean backwards.

Variation: To allow ease of movement underneath your heel and front of back foot, try placing a couple of towels underneath or something that will allow you to slide slowly with control as you deepen. It is important that you remember to always stay in control of the posture, therefore use your hands for support and deepen the posture slowly. Be patient with yourself.

Cave Entering Posture

ท่าเข้าคูหา

Tha = Posture; *Khao* = Entering; *Khuha* = Cave

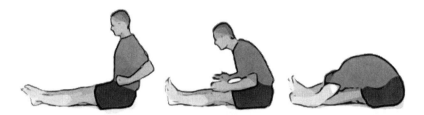

Preparation: Sit with legs out straight, lengthen your spine and draw your turned fists into the side of your waist.

Movement: Fold forwards at the hips and at the same time, rotate and open your fists as you reach forwards. Aim to get your chest to your knees and head to shins. Complete the movement by returning to the preparation position.

Focus: Lengthen your upper body.

Active Form: Continuous flow.

Passive Form: Train the edge on the low.

Inhale: Return.

Exhale: Enter the cave.

Channel and Intensify Life Force: Draw energy in as you create fists. Feel your body sink down as you soften your back and the back of your legs. Focus on energy going through the top of your head and behind your sitting bones.

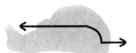

Purpose:
Muscular Area: Back of body including back of legs / Core-abs and back.
Benefit: Nervous system / Internal organs / Squeezing on the low increases the flow of life force to your abdominal organs / Directs your awareness inwards / Balances life force / Creating fists strengthens the flow of life force / Stress reliever / Letting go.

Self-Defence: Freedom to move in kicks and knees at different heights / Helps with the fist rotation in straight punches / Rotating the fist adds velocity, giving the punch more power.

Interest: The aim is to eventually squeeze your body together as though going through a tight gap in a cave. The deeper you go into the pose, the less you will be able to see and so the more you will need to direct your awareness inwards.

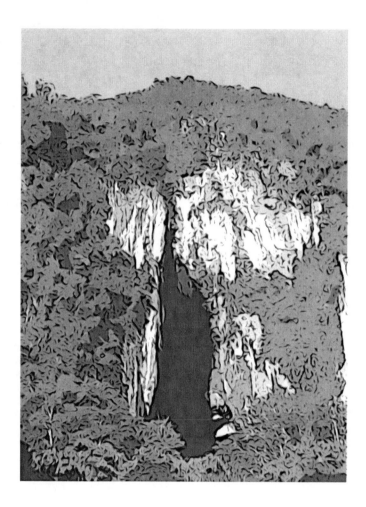

Salute Earth Posture

ท่าชมพสุธา

Tha = Posture; *Chom* = Salute; *Phasutha* = Earth

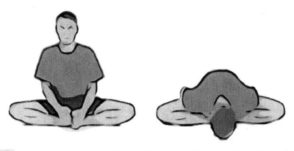

Preparation: Sit with the soles of your feet together and heels in close. Lengthen your spine.

Movement: Lower your knees followed by lowering your head to the earth.

Focus: Lengthen your upper body. Stay soft to help you connect to the earth.

Active Form: Raise legs or head up and down.

Passive Form: Train the edge on the low.

Inhale: As you rise / Lengthen spine

Exhale: As you lower.

Channel and Intensify Life Force: Forms a circuit of life force within your body. Energy opening and flowing down through your knees. Energy also goes through the top of your head as you lengthen the spine.

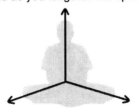

Purpose:
Muscular Area: Ankles / Knees / Hips / Inner thighs / Core-abs and back.
Benefit: Can help make the meditation posture (p.34) more comfortable / Opens out pelvic area / Kidneys / Prostate gland.
Self-Defence: Round kicks and round knees.

Interest: Also known as Hermit Relaxing Posture.

Tri Worship Posture

ท่าไตรบูชา

Tha = Posture; ***Trai*** = Tri; ***Bucha*** = Worship

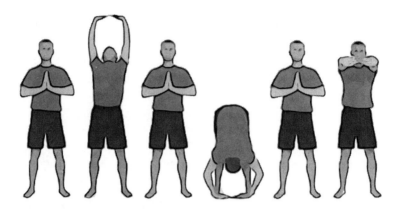

Preparation: Stand in a shoulder width stance and raise your hands into a *wai*.

Movement: The posture has three parts to it. Firstly, reach your palms to the sky and return to the *wai* position. Secondly, fold forward from your hips to reach your palms to the earth and return to the *wai* position. Thirdly, reach your palms forward and return to the *wai* position. Repeat.

Focus: Maintain softness in your shoulders. This posture works very well if you visualize pushing against something to help channel your energy.

Active Form: Continuous flow synchronized with the breath.

Passive Form: All three parts can be trained at the edge.

Inhale: Return to *wai*.

Exhale: As you reach.

Channel and Intensify Life Force: On all three movements, as you push your palms away, energy radiates from the core, through the palms and beyond.

Purpose:
Muscular Area: Back of legs / Shoulders.
Benefit: Regulates all the internal organs / Combats fatigue / Posture of back and shoulders / Flow of life force to core-abs and back / Balance energy / Releases tension.
Self-Defence: Practise the *wai* movement. Get into a good habit of returning to a guard position after an attack or defence movement.

Interest: The meaning of Tri in this name is to worship Buddhism's Three Gems by way of *Wai*.

The Three Gems are:
- Buddha (enlightened or awakened one).
- His teachings (path to enlightenment).
- Practising monks.

Cave Guarding Posture

ท่าเฝ้าคูหา

Tha = Posture; *Fao* = Guarding; *Khuha* = Cave

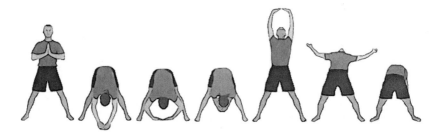

Preparation: Stand in a wide stance and raise your hands into a *wai*.

Movement: The posture consists of five parts. Firstly, fold at your hips to reach down and in front. Secondly, reach straight down. Thirdly, reach under and behind the legs. Fourthly, rise up and reach upwards. Lastly, reach backwards by bending your knees and arching your back. Complete the posture by returning your hands to the *wai* position. Repeat.

Focus: Maintain softness in your shoulders. Reach far so that all parts of the cave are guarded.

Active Form: Continuous flow synchronized with your breath.

Passive Form: All five parts can be trained at the edge.

Inhale: As you release.

Exhale: As you reach.

Channel and Intensify Life Force: As you reach your hands away on each part, energy radiates from your core, through your fingertips and beyond.

Purpose:
Muscular Area: Back and front of body / Backs of legs / Inner thighs / Core-abs and back.
Benefit: Release tension and express freedom of movement in both sides of body / Connect with and reverse the effects of gravity / Calming / Same effects as forward and back bends.
Self-Defence: Agility in defence and attack.

Star and Moon
Accompanying Posture

ท่าคลอเคล้าดาวเดือน

Tha = Posture; *Khlo* = Accompanying; *Khlao* = To Mingle Together (To Roll);
Dao = Star; *Duean* = Moon

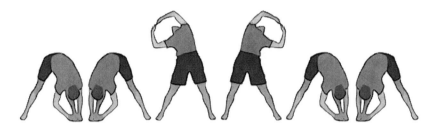

Preparation: Stand in a wide stance with your hands in a *wai* position.

Movement: Fold at the hips and with both hands reach down to one foot, then continue to go all the way round until you reach the opposite foot. Change direction and repeat.

Focus: Push your hips forward when arching back.

Active Form: Continuous movement.

Inhale: First half of the posture, as you rise.

Exhale: Second half of the posture, as you lower.

Channel and Intensify Life Force: Energy radiates from your core, through your hands and beyond as you rotate round.

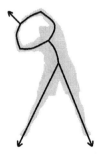

Purpose:
Muscular Area: Back of legs / Inner thighs / Core-abs and back.
Benefit: Release tension and express the freedom of movement in the core-abs and back / Connect with and reverse the effects of gravity / Calming.
Self-Defence: Agility in defence and attack.

Interest: Ancient Thai warriors understood that the stars and the moon spun round a central point. They were aware that they needed to unite with all and be connected with everything in the universe.

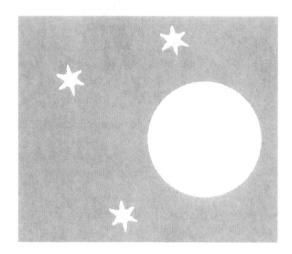

Wai Postures
ท่าไหว้

Tha = Posture; *Wai* = Respectful Thai Gesture

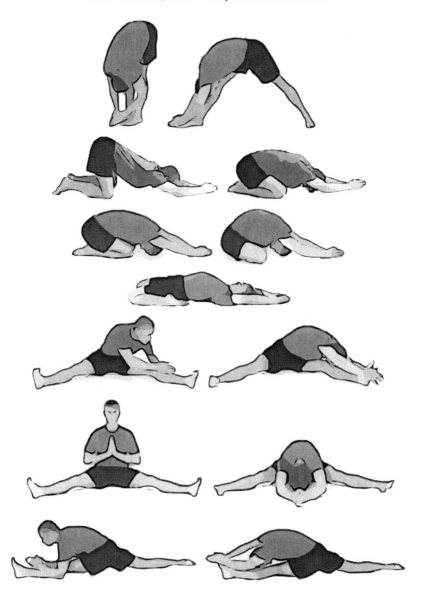

Preparation: Bring your palms together to raise the energy to your heart.

Movement: This is an advanced series of postures where the hands are kept in a *wai* position.

Focus: Extending you energy outwards through the *wai* and beyond.

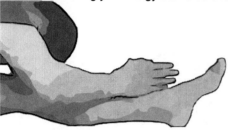

Active Form: Continuous movement.

Passive Form: Train at the edges.

Inhale: As you return.   **Exhale:** As you stretch and reach.

Channel and Intensify Life Force: Extend and reach the *wai* in the direction you intend to channel your life force.

Purpose:
Muscular Area: Mainly the back of the body.
Benefit: Energy to your heart / Compassion.
Self-Defence: *Wai* guard / *Wai* strikes / *Wai* blocks / *Wai* locks and breaks.

Interest: The *wai* is a respectful greeting in Thailand. All of Muay's defence and attack techniques can flow easily from the *wai* position. It forms an excellent protective guard which you can feel safe behind and it also forms many weapons that can be used to defend or attack. It has the ability to create a fascinating oneness with your opponent. The higher the *wai* and the more you *wai*, the greater the respect you are giving your enemy. The greater your enemy's attack, the greater you show respect for them with a higher *wai* guard and more *wai* strikes.

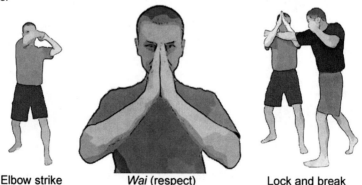

Elbow strike   *Wai* (respect)   Lock and break

Core-Abs and Back

God of Air / Wind Clears and Brightens Posture

ท่าผ่องแผ้วพระพาย

Tha = Posture; *Phong Phaeo* = Clears and Brightens;
Phra Phai = God of Air / Wind

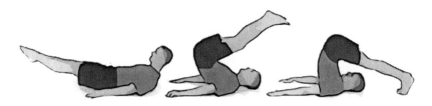

Preparation: Lie on your back, feet close together with arms at your side.

Movement: Raise your legs, shoulders and head slightly off the ground. Keep your lower back close to the ground. Then raise your feet up and over your head. When you return keep your feet off the ground and then repeat.

Focus: Keep your legs extended.

Active Form: Continuous movement, keeping your feet, shoulders and head off the ground upon return.

Passive Form: Train the edge when your feet are over your head.

Inhale: Raise feet up / As you return.   **Exhale:** Bring your feet over your head.

Channel and Intensify Life Force: Dynamic opposition of the finger tips and heels. A line of energy also travels up through torso.

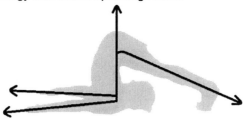

Purpose:
Muscular Area: Back of body / Back of legs / Core-abs and back / Spine / Shoulders / Neck.
Benefit: Nourishes spinal nerves / Flow of life force to neck and spine / Thyroid gland / Digestion / Releases tension / Directs your awareness inwards / Boosts energy.

Self-Defence: Part of developing a balanced powerful core for all defence and attack techniques / Helps you to deal with strikes to your abdominals / Improves breathing and ability to soften during grappling, which can be stressful and uncomfortable due to pressure up close to the chest / Kicks.

Interest: Phra Phai is the god of air/wind and father of Hanuman (great white monkey). Knowledge of the breath of life *(Lom Haichai)* is believed to have been passed from Phra Phai to his son who went on to share this knowledge with many others.

Hanuman can be revived by the passing wind. In following with this belief, it has become a tradition for masters to blow over a Muay warrior's head before going into battle.

Wat Arun in Bangkok.
Prangs around the temple represent the four major oceans.
Each contain statues of the air/wind God on horseback.

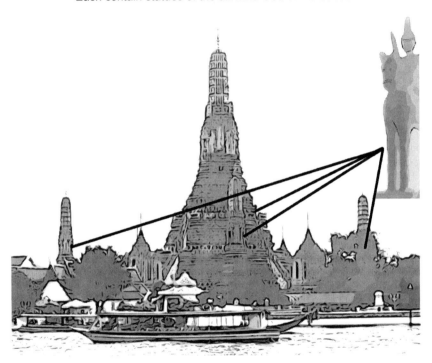

Variation: Support your back with your hands if you cannot lower your feet to the ground.

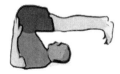

Hermit Crushes
Medicine Posture

ท่าฤๅษีบดยา

Tha = Posture; *Ruesi* = Hermit; *Bot* = Crushes; *Ya* = Medicine

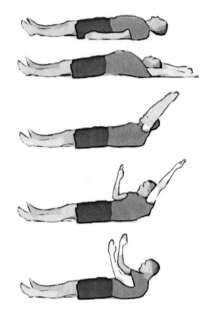

Preparation: Lie on your back with your feet hip width apart and your arms behind your head.

Movement: Curl up with your shoulders, head and arms off the ground, then apply two downwards elbow strikes in quick succession, targeting your abdominals. As you return, raise your arms right back behind your head and repeat.

Focus: As you curl up, maintain a distance of a fist between your chin and your chest. Keep your lower back close to the ground.

Active Form: Continuous movement.

Inhale: Lower and raise your arms behind head.

Exhale: As you squeeze up and elbow strike.

Channel and Intensify Life Force: The important line of aliveness comes from your centre, travels up through your straight arm and way beyond your fingertips. Be contraction free in your lower body to connect to the earth.

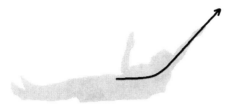

Purpose:

Muscular Area: Core-abs.

Benefit: Beautiful waist line / Natural postural support.

Self-Defence: Part of developing a balanced, powerful core for all defence and attack techniques / Helps you to deal with strikes to your abdominals / Elbows / Covers and opens.

Interest: There is also a master trick with the same name which forms an attack pattern of repeated elbow strikes. For example, a repeated combination of downward elbow strikes targeting your opponent's head or collar bone, or an elbow thrust targeting the opponent's neck followed by an uppercut elbow targeting their chin.

Interest: The posture mimics the action of a Thai hermit crushing medicine with a pestle and mortar. Hermits were renowned for their wisdom in medicine and healing.

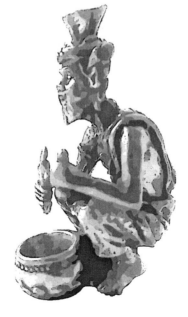

Surging Wave Wind Posture

ท่าผวาคลื่นลม

Tha = Posture; *Phawa* = Fright, Rush in (Surging);
Khluen = Wave; *Lom* = Wind

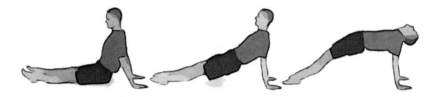

Preparation: Sit with your legs extended, hip width apart. Place your hands slightly behind you, shoulder width apart. Spread your fingers wide and point them away from you.

Movement: Raise your hips, expand your chest and if possible relax your head back. Then return to the preparation position and repeat.

Focus: Powerful lift that opens up the front of your body.

Active Form: Continuous up and down movement or hold on the high.

Inhale: As you rise.

Exhale: As you lower.

Channel and Intensify Life Force: Visualize energy flowing through your hips and high up to the sky. As you lift you can also tune into the dynamic opposition from your toes through to the top of your head.

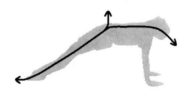

Purpose:
Muscular Area: Front of body / Hips / Core-abs and back / Shoulders / Arms / Wrists.
Benefit: Pelvis control / Part of developing a balanced firm core for excellent posture / Opens up chest.
Self-Defence: Faith and confidence even when you are most open and vulnerable / Helps with the thrusting movement of the hips in push kicks and knee strikes / Elbows.

Interest: Feel the difference it makes when you visualize a wave rising up from underneath you, so that your body lifts up effortlessly and you only contract the muscles that you need. If you struggle to feel the difference, start by doing a few with all your muscles contracted. You can also visualize wind energy filling your body as it opens up.

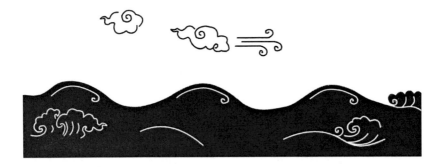

Variation: An easier option is to bend your knees.

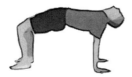

Arrow Posture

ท่าลูกศร

Tha = Posture; *Luk Son* = Arrow

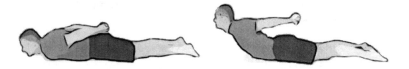

Preparation: Lie on your front and keep your feet together. Interlock your fingers behind your back.

Movement: Lift your head, shoulders and chest off the ground, drawing your arms back at the same time.

Focus: Maintain softness in your legs and backside. Keep your palms together.

Active Form: Continuous up and down or train the edge on the high.

Inhale: As you rise.

Exhale: As you lower.

Channel and Intensify Life Force: Energy rises upwards along your spine and through the top of your head. Your shoulders are pulled back and down as energy flows through your arms and beyond your hands.

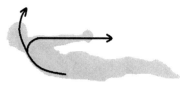

Purpose:
Muscular Area: Lower back / Spine.
Benefit: Part of developing a balanced firm core for excellent posture / Relieves tension in mid back, upper back and shoulders / Combats rounded shoulders / Opens up chest / Also has same benefits as back bends.
Self-Defence: Part of developing a balanced powerful core for all defence and attack techniques.

Variation: Bend from side to side on the high.

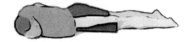

72

Bow Posture

ท่าคันศร

Tha = Posture; *Khan Son* = Bow

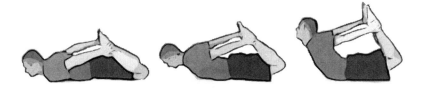

Preparation: Lie on your front and grab your ankles, keeping your feet and knees hip width apart.

Movement: Simultaneously raise your upper and lower body off the ground. Lower and repeat.

Focus: Feel your feet push against your hands as you draw yourself up to gain range.

Active Form: Continuous movement of drawing your body up and down.

Passive Form: Train the range as you pull upwards.

Inhale: As you draw the bow.

Exhale: As you lower / As you draw the bow further.

Channel and Intensify Life Force: Energy extends through your head and your toes.

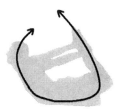

Purpose:
Muscular Area: Front of body / Front of thighs and hips / Spine / Back / Shoulders.
Benefit: Part of developing a balanced firm core for excellent posture / Digestion / Encourages full natural breaths / Vitality / Combat laziness.
Self-Defence: Gain more movement for loading up weapons, for example, straight knees in grappling.

Serpent Snake with a Crystal in its Mouth Posture

ท่านาคาคาบแก้ว

Tha = Posture; *Nak* = Serpent Snake *(Naga)*; *Khap* = Holds in Mouth; *Kaeo* = Crystal

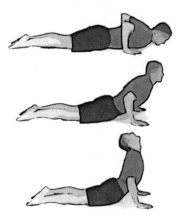

Preparation: Lie on to your front with your hands beside your chest and your fingers spread out wide.

Movement: Curl your head, chest and abdominals up off the ground and open your mouth. Lower and repeat.

Focus: Maintain softness to allow your hips to stay rooted to the ground.

Active Form: Continuous flow up and down.

Passive Form: Train the edge on the arch back.

Inhale: As you push up and open.

Exhale: As you elongate the spine / As you lower.

Channel and Intensify Life Force: Feel the life force rising as your chest pushes forwards and your spine bends. Your shoulders stay down as your energy pushes through your hands and deep into the earth. Stay rooted to the earth by drawing your hips down and be contraction free in the lower body.

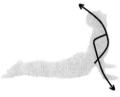

Purpose:
Muscular Area: Spine / Core-abs and back.
Benefit: Abdominal organs / Release tension in back / Flow of energy to spine / Nerves / Opens Chest / Energise / Concentration / Posture / Confidence.
Self-Defence: Part of developing a balanced powerful core for all defence and attack techniques / Evasion.

Interest: The crystal is believed to immortalize Naga. When Thai masters talk about immortality, they do not mean living forever but that you live your full optimum life free of disease, illness, injury and surviving battles. There is a familiar saying that you are as young as your spine is supple.

The latissimus dorsi muscles (lats) of the back can be activated to form the hood like shape of Naga. The serpent snake would rise up like a cobra if threatened. It is important to have an attitude like a snake, defensive, not aggressive.

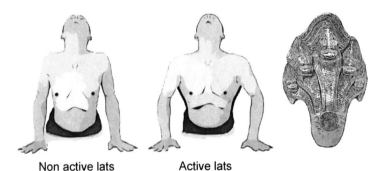

Non active lats   Active lats

The picture in the centre shows the elbows wide to allow you to see the movement, but when you do it ensure to keep the elbows in.

Variation: An easier option is to rise up from your forearms rather than your hands.

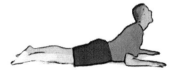

Hermits Cross Twist Posture

ท่าฤๅษีบิดข้าม

Tha = Posture; ***Ruesi*** = Hermits; ***Bit*** = Twist; ***Kham*** = Cross

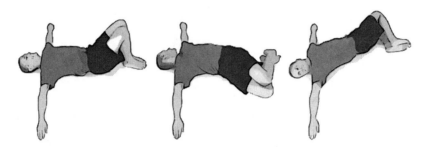

Preparation: Lie on your back with your knees bent and spread your arms out to your side.

Movement: Roll your knees from side to side and as your knees go to one side, turn your head in the opposite direction. Repeat from side to side.

Focus: Keep your shoulders and arms on the ground.

Active Form: Continuous movement from side to side.

Passive Form: Train the edge on the low.

Inhale: As you lengthen spine / As you return.

Exhale: As you twist.

Channel and Intensify Life Force: Generate energy by twisting your spine. Your spine must stay lengthened. Twisting wrings out negative energy.

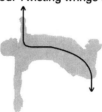

Purpose:
Muscular Area: Outer thighs / Buttocks / Hips / Core-abs and back / Spine / Neck.
Benefit: Agility in back / Releases tension in back / Opens up chest / Spinal nerves / Digestion / Increases flow of life force / Invigorates spine / Opens and unblocks various *sen* lines / Refreshes.

Self-Defence: Adaptable and agile in defence and attack / Extra power from the core in defence and attack movements.

Variation: There are many different ways to practise the twist as illustrated below.

Raise your feet off the ground and twist from side to side.

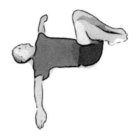

Extend one leg and just bring one knee over to the side. Use your hand to assist. This is an ideal way to practise the posture in a passive way.

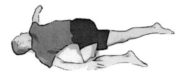

Twist with legs straight.

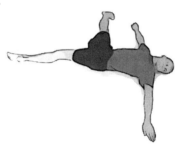

Or a seated twist.

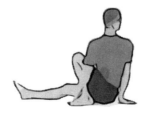

Giant Turns Posture

ท่ายักษ์เหลียวหลัง

Tha = Posture; *Yak* = Giant; *Liao Lang* = Turns

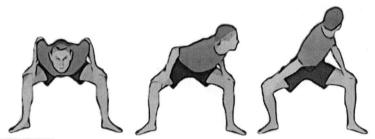

Preparation: Stand in a shoulder width stance with your knees bent at 90 degrees with your hands on top of your knees.

Movement: Fold forward from your hips then twist round and continue up to the side. Then stay low as you twist round to the other side. Repeat.

Focus: Extending and twisting your spine.

Active Form: Continuous movement from side to side.

Passive Form: Train the edge on the twist.

Inhale: Return to centre.

Exhale: Twist round.

Channel and Intensify Life Force: Generate energy by twisting your spine. Wring out negative energy. Gently pushing against your knee will increase the twist.

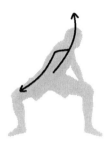

Purpose:

Muscular Area: Legs / Buttocks / Spine.

Benefit: Posture / Agility in lower back / Spinal nerves / Flow of life force to spine / Releases tension in spine / Internal organs / Digestion / Relieves heat and stress of heart / Refreshes / Increases life force.

Self-Defence: Agility in spine.

Interest: Even the many giant demons have a positive side. Statues of giants can be seen in Thai temples where they act as protective guardians.

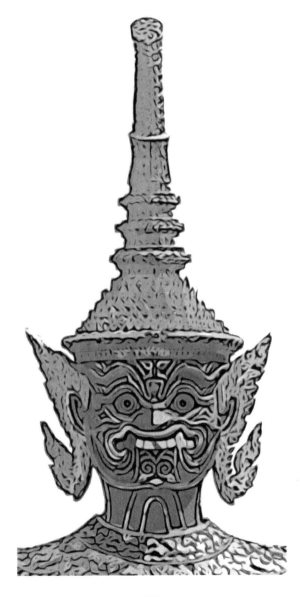

Mountain Hiding Posture

ท่าพรางขุนเขา

Tha = Posture; *Phrang* = Hiding; *Khun Khao* = Mountain

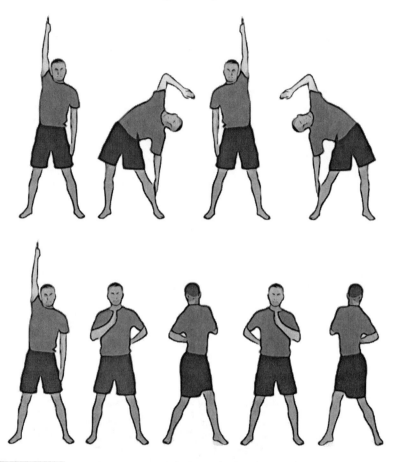

Preparation: Stand in a shoulder width stance, knees soft.

Movement: The posture consists of two parts. Firstly, reach your arm up through the midline of your body and then bend over to the side. Aim to increase the range three times. Complete both sides. Secondly, raise your arm high and drop it down to form a single *wai*, then twist your body round to the opposite side. Again, aim to increase the range three times. Repeat on opposite side to complete the sequence.

For details about the *wai* see p.64 and p.150.

Focus: Use the breath as you train the edge three times.

Active Form: Continuous flow from side to side.

Passive Form: At the edge of both parts of the posture.

Inhale: To return.

Exhale: Bend / Twist.

Channel and Intensify Life Force: Radiating from your core, through your finger tips and beyond.

Purpose of Part One (Side Bend):
Muscular Area: Side of torso / Back / Neck.
Benefit: Agility in spine / Spinal Nerves / Decompress spine / Digestion / Removes excess heat from heart / Increase flow of energy / Release tension and stress / Posture / Tones respiratory muscles / Focus / Determination.
Self-Defence: Helps you practise a master trick called Old Monk Holding Up Gourd (a type of vegetable). The technique is used to defend against punches by raising the arm high to divert your opponent's punch, which opens them up and enables you to protect the side of your head / The movement can also prepare you for loading up downward elbow strikes / Side bends help you to lean your body weight in on round kicks / Covering and opening.

Purpose of Part Two (Twist):
Muscular Area: Core-abs and back / Neck.
Benefit: Agility in spine / Invigorates spine / Opens up chest / Nervous system / Digestion / Eye focus / Release tension and stress / Increase flow of energy / Refreshing.
Self-Defence: Forms a powerful defensive upper inner brush (Brushing the Nose) / Swiping / Turning your whole body as one with swing punches and elbows for added power.

Upper

Swan Flies in Air Posture

ท่าหงส์เหิน

Tha = Posture; *Hong* = Swan; *Hoen* = Fly in the Air

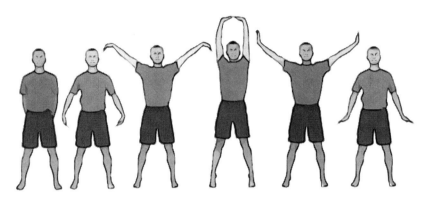

Preparation: Stand in a shoulder width stance with your hands behind your back. Have your palms facing upwards with fingertips touching.

Movement: Spread your arms out wide and bring above your head with your wrists relaxed. As you reach high, turn your palms up to the sky. Pull your hands back as you lower to the preparation position and repeat.

Focus: Keep your shoulders back and down and draw your wings back throughout the movement.

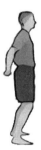

Active Form: Continuous movement.

Inhale: As you spread your wings above.

Exhale: As you lower.

Channel and Intensify Life Force: From your heart, through your finger tips and through the air. Stay rooted to the earth by being contraction free in the lower body.

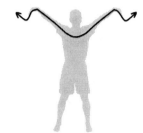

Purpose:
Muscular Area: Upper back.
Benefit: Stimulates heart / Clears and calms the mind / Connection with breath.
Self-Defence: Power in grappling / Elbows / Trapping.

Interest: Mimics the movement of a swan flying freely in the air.

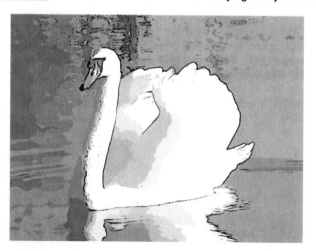

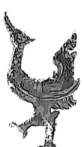

Variation: The movement can also be practised by lifting one heel up behind so you stand on one leg. This will help improve balance and eye focus with soft gaze.

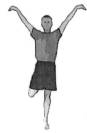

Breath Moving Posture

ท่าเดินลมปราณ

Tha = Posture; *Doen* = Moving; *Lom Pran* = Breath

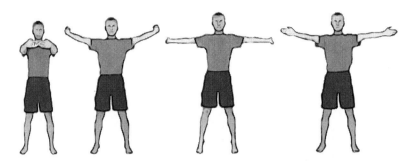

Preparation: Stand in a shoulder width stance with your arms extended out in front of you. Have your palms facing you and your fingertips close together.

Movement: Draw your arms back keeping your palms facing towards you, whilst simultaneously lifting your heels high. As you return, draw your hands back so that your palms face away from you whilst lowering your heels. Repeat.

Focus: Keep your shoulders down. Absorb life force on the in breath.

Active Form: Continuous movement.

Passive Form: Train the edge when your arms are open wide.

Inhale: Open arms and lift heels.

Exhale: Close arms and lower heels.

Channel and Intensify Life Force: Tune into the dynamic opposition when you spread your arms out wide. When you are wide open, feel the energy that travels through your fingertips, into the air and afar. As you bring your hands close feel the energy connect between your fingertips. Energy out, energy in.

Purpose:
Muscular Area: Upper back / Back of shoulders.
Benefit: Opens up chest / Posture / Eye focus with soft gaze / Focus / Connection with breath / Balance.
Self-Defence: It develops power for the strike techniques called Monkey Swings Revered Sword (p.172) and Prepare for Battle (p.174) / It helps with advanced ways of doing techniques simultaneously, for example, blocking a punch by brushing it inwards and striking with a swing punch inwards at the same time / Helps posture in grappling / Improves balance in footwork when your heels are high / Elbows.

King Draws Back Bow and Arrow Posture

ท่าพระรามน้าวศร

Tha = Posture; *Phra Ram* = King Rama; *Nao* = Draws Back Bow;
Son = Arrow

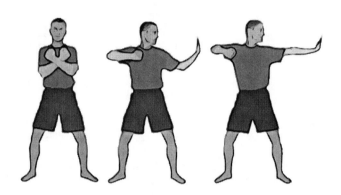

Preparation: Stand in a wide stance with your arms crossed in a guard position called a Thousand Fists.

Movement: Extend your lead arm with your hand pulled back and simultaneously draw your other fist back with the elbow raised, turning your head in the direction of aim. Continue the movement by changing your guard and repeating on the other side. If you aim to the left side you need to use a right guard, with your right fist behind the left. Remember to change the guard as you alternate from side to side.

Focus: A great opportunity to experience and feel the life force in your fingertips as your draw your extended hand back.

Active Form: Alternate from side to side.

Passive Form: Train the edge on the draw back.

Inhale: As you draw back the bow.

Exhale: As you release the arrow and return.

Channel and Intensify Life Force: Drawing the bow draws in energy. Visualize the action as you push your palm against the bow, whilst your elbow draws back as you pull the bowstring. Stay rooted to the earth by being contraction free in the lower body.

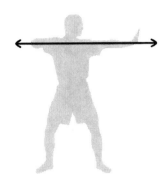

Purpose:
Muscular Area: Upper back / Back of shoulders / Neck.
Benefit: Heart / Lungs / Circulation / Small intestine / Release tension in shoulders, upper back and neck / Focus.
Self-Defence: The movement is practised in the *Wai Khru* and a master trick. For the master trick, pull back the attacking arm at the same time as blocking outwards and so loading up your strike to follow / This is great way to create extra power. Energy out, energy in / Shielding and opening.

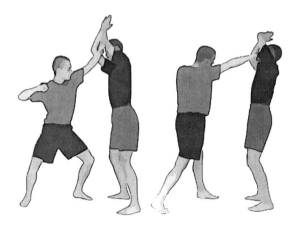

Interest: The king is called Rama who is the hero in the Ramakien story. The bow is one of King Rama's main weapons. According to the legend, King Rama went hunting for a deer that his wife Sida desired. Using his bow and arrow he hits the deer on his third shot. Meanwhile, back at King Rama's palace, Princess Sida is abducted by the giant demon Tosakanth. The deer turns out to be a giant demon called Mareet, who was carrying orders from his relative Tosakanth to transform himself into a deer to trick King Rama away from the palace and so leaving Sida unprotected.

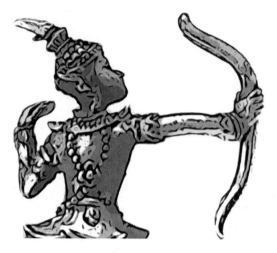

Variation: The movement can also be practised by lifting one heel up behind you so you are standing on one leg. This will help with balance and eye focus with soft gaze.

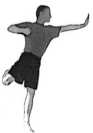

Variation: It is also possible to extend both arms at the same time.

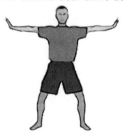

Open Heart Posture

ท่าเผยดวงใจ

Tha = Posture; *Phoei* = Open; *Duangchai* = Heart

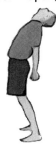

Preparation: Stand in a wide stance with your fingers interlocked behind your back.

Movement: Arch back and draw your hands down.

Focus: Keep your shoulders down and palms together.

Passive Form: Train the edge by drawing the hands downwards.

Inhale: As you open.

Exhale: As you deepen / As you lengthen and arch back.

Channel and Intensify Life Force: Energy radiates from the heart as your chest pushes forwards and your spine bends. Keep your shoulders down as your energy pushes through your hands. Stay rooted to the earth by being contraction free in the lower body.

Purpose:
Muscular Area: Back / Chest / Front of shoulders.
Benefit: Abdominal organs / Release tension in back / Flow of life force to spine / Opens up chest / Posture / Concentration.
Self-Defence: Grappling posture.

Interest: Opening your heart with compassion is vital in achieving happiness and oneness.

Variation: Draw your hands up and back away from your body.

Reverse Wai Posture

ท่าไหว้กลับหลัง

Tha = Posture; *Wai* = Wai; *Klap Lang* = Reverse

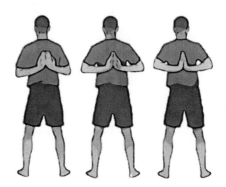

Preparation: Stand in a wide stance with your hands in a *wai* behind your back.

Movement: Draw your elbows inwards and raise the *wai*.

Focus: Keep your shoulders down and palms together.

Passive Form: Train the edge.

Inhale: Open your chest.

Exhale: Bring elbows inwards and soften shoulders.

Channel and Intensify Life Force: The energy comes alive as you bring the palms together and raise the *wai* up the spine. The main focus is bringing your elbows inwards. Stay rooted to the earth by being contraction free in the lower body.

Purpose:
Muscular Area: Chest / Front of shoulders / Arms / Elbows / Wrists.
Benefit: Posture / Helps improve low moods or depression.
Self-Defence: Grappling posture / Elbows / Locks and breaks.

Enjoyment Bringing Posture

ท่าพาเพลิดเพลิน

Tha = Posture; *Pha* = Bringing; *Phloet Phloen* = Enjoyment

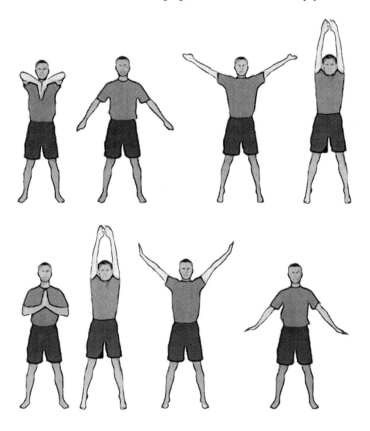

Preparation: Stand in a shoulder width stance with the backs of your hands together in downward *wai*.

Movement: This posture consists of two parts. First, completely rotate both your arms forwards. As you raise your arms also raise your heels off the ground and turn your palms. When you lower your arms also lower your heels. Repeat as many times as you need. Secondly, with hands in a *wai*, completely rotate both your arms backwards. This time turn your palms as you lower your arms. As before, raise your heels up and down in sync with the arms.

Focus: Keep your shoulders down. Full wide rotations with your arms.

Active Form: Continuous movement.

Inhale: As you raise arms and heels.

Exhale: As you lower arms and heels.

Channel and Intensify Life Force: Energy radiating around and afar in a wide circle. It travels straight through your fingertips and beyond.

Purpose:
Muscular Area: Upper back / Back of shoulders.
Benefit: Opens up chest / Posture / Eye focus with soft gaze / Connection with breath / Refresh / Balance.
Self-Defence: Grappling posture / Locks and breaks / Swipes, blocks, opens and covers / Elbows / See p.27 and p.29 for details on how it can be used in battle.

Interest: This movement is similar to a combination of the postures called Elephant Destroying the Holding Pen and Tiger Destroying the Hunter's Tree Hide. In the Enjoyment Bringing Posture, there is a much wider range of movement and the heels should always be raised and lowered as described.

Body Rides the Waves Posture

ท่าเคลื่อนกายใต้คลื่น

Tha = Posture; *Khluean* = Moving; *Kai* = Body; *To Khluen* = Against Wave

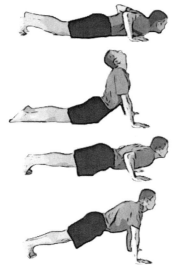

Preparation: Lie on to your front with your hands beside your chest and your fingers spread out wide.

Movement: This posture consists of two parts. Firstly, curl your head, shoulders, abdominals and hips off the ground, then lower. Secondly, tuck your toes under and complete a push-up. Then repeat.

Focus: Create a flowing movement throughout the posture.

Active Form: Continuous movement.

Passive Form: Train the edge on the first part.

Inhale: As you arch back.

Exhale: As you rise up in push up.

Channel and Intensify Life Force: Use the visualization of a wave underneath your body to help you push up in both parts.

Muscular Area: Spine / Core-abs and back / Back of arms / Front of shoulders / Chest / Wrists.

Benefit: Opens Chest / Vitality / Same effect on the body as back bends and push-ups.

Self-Defence: Punch power / Elbows / Locks and breaks / Evasion and deflection.

Interest: Feel the difference it makes when you visualize flowing with an oncoming wave. Let go and only contract the muscles you need. If you struggle to feel the difference, start by doing a few with all your muscles tense and contracted.

Variation: Instead of a sequence, you can practise each part individually.

Half-Serpent Snake, Half-Crocodile Posture

ท่าเหรา

Tha = Posture; *Haera* = Half-Serpent Snake Half-Crocodile / Dragon

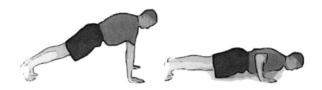

Preparation: Push up position with your hands underneath your shoulders, tuck your toes under and extend your legs.

Movement: The posture has two parts to it. Firstly, all you need to do is hold the preparation position. Secondly, bend your elbows to lower so that your body is just off the ground. Hold that position and then push yourself back up to the first position and repeat.

Focus: Lengthen your body throughout the posture. Maintain the natural curves in your spine.

Active Form: Hold on the high and on the low.

Inhale: As you lower.

Exhale: As you push up.

Inhale and Exhale: Natural breath movement as you hold the positions.

Channel and Intensify Life Force: Once you have lengthened your body, you can then increase intensity by visualizing energy channelling through your arms, hands and deep into the earth. You can increase ease and softness to the posture by imagining you are buoyant in water.

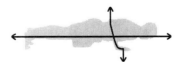

Purpose:
Muscular Area: Core-abs and back / Front of shoulders / Chest / Back of arms.
Benefit: Posture / Patience through challenging times / Pad holding.

Self-Defence: Punch power / Part of developing a balanced powerful core for all defence and attack techniques / Blocking.

Interest: Thai mythology is abundant with diverse, mysterious and magical creatures. They are believed to live in the Himaphan Forest located in the Himalayas, a place that is invisible to mere mortals.

Many of the creatures feature in the story of the Ramakien.

One of the wonderful dragon-like creatures is called Haera who is half-serpent snake, half-crocodile. Haera's amphibious nature is demonstrated in this posture, on land when posture high, in water when posture low.

The qualities of Haera are patience and stillness. This can be seen when watching a crocodile hunt. With these qualities, we can often gain greater results in the postures.

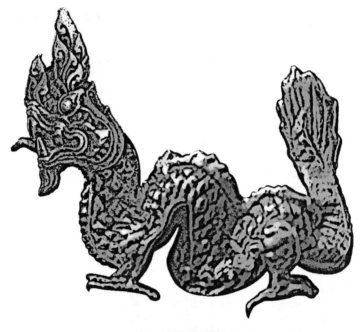

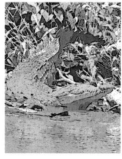

Muaythai Push-up
and Knee Block

มวยไทยดันพื้น และ สกัด เข่า

Muaythai = Muaythai; *Dan Phuen* = Push-up; *Lae* = and; *Sakat* = Block;
Khao = Knee

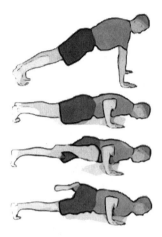

Preparation: Push-up position with your hands underneath your shoulders, tuck your toes under and extend your legs.

Movement: Bend your elbows to go into a low push-up position and then raise your knee to form a knee block. Complete both sides and push back up. Repeat.

Focus: Lengthen your body throughout the posture.

Active Form: Continuous flow.

Inhale: As you lower.

Exhale: As you push up / As you knee block.

Channel and Intensify Life Force: Once your body is lengthened, the main focus is to increase softness and save energy by visualizing a giant helping you by pulling you upwards. You can increase the intensity by pressing deep into the earth.

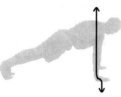

Purpose:
Muscular Area: Hips / Core-abs and back / Chest / Front of shoulders / Back of arms.
Benefit: Increase metabolic rate / Bone density / Pad holding / Coordination.
Self-Defence: Knee blocks / Punches / Elbows / Grappling / Blocking / Shielding.

Interest: Feel the difference it makes when you visualize a giant pulling you up so that you only contract the muscles you need. If you struggle to feel the difference, start by doing a few with all your muscles contracted.

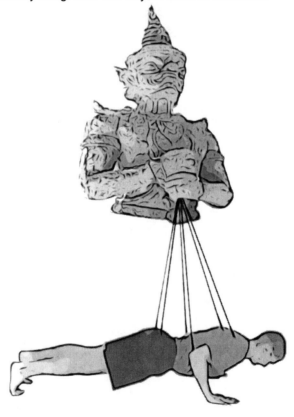

Muaythai Push-up
and Knee Slap

มวยไทยดันพื้น และ ตบเข่า

Muaythai = Muaythai; ***Dan Phuen*** = Push-up; ***Lae*** = and; ***Top*** = Slap;
Khao = Knee

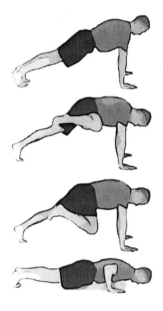

Preparation: Push-up position with your hands underneath your shoulders, tuck your toes under and extend your legs.

Movement: Raise your knee outwards to the side then slap your knee inwards. Do the other side and then lower and rise up to complete a push-up. Repeat.

Focus: The knee slap entails rotating the hip slightly so that you lead with your knee. Lengthen your body throughout the posture.

Active Form: Continuous flow.

Inhale: As you lower.

Exhale: As you push up / As you knee slap.

Channel and Intensify Life Force: Once your body is lengthened the main focus is to increase softness and save energy by visualizing a giant helping you by pulling you upwards.

Purpose:

Muscular Area: Hips / Core-abs and back / Chest / Front of shoulders / Back of arms.

Benefit: Awareness of the freedom of movement in hip / Flow of life force to pelvic area / Increase metabolic rate / Bone density / Pad holding.

Self-Defence: Knee Slaps / Punches / Elbows / Grappling / Blocking.

Interest: All the Muay push-ups require you to be able to lift around 75 per cent of your body weight. This makes it a challenging movement and ideal for gaining strength.

Muaythai Push-up

มวยไทยดันพื้น

Muaythai = Muaythai; *Dan Phuen* = Push-up

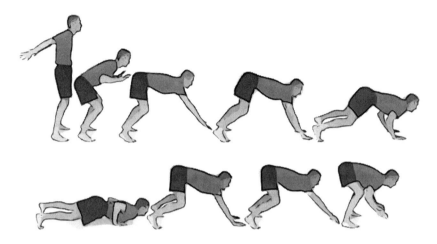

Preparation: Stand in a wide stance, knees slightly bent.

Movement: Clap your hands behind your back. Bend your knees to drop down into a push-up position. To help absorb your landing keep your elbows soft and land with your fingers spread wide. Continue to bend your elbows, going into a low push-up position, then push up with the help of your legs to return to the preparation position. Repeat.

Focus: Aim to land like a feather and use an explosive movement to spring back up.

Active Form: Continuous flow.

Inhale: As you clap and drop down into the low push-up.

Exhale: As you push back up.

Channel and Intensify Life Force: The main focus is to increase softness and save energy by visualizing a giant helping you by pulling you upwards.

Purpose:
Muscular Area: Abdominals / Chest / Front of shoulders / Back of arms / Wrists.
Benefit: Gain explosive power / Response time / Increase metabolic rate / Bone density / Pad holding.

Self-Defence: Punches / Elbows / Grappling / Blocking / Catching and shielding / Extra power for the techniques called Repel the Tiger (p.170) and Tiger Claws (p.178).

Interest: The modern Thai army practise many push-ups. They do it with their heads up, looking forwards, to create a habit of being able to see their enemy at all times.

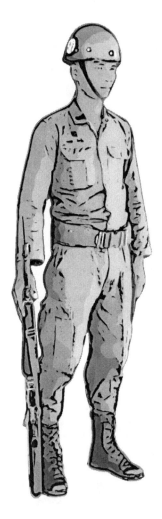

Variation: To increase the challenge you can also add the following: complete a push-up and instead of springing back up to a standing position, spring up and clap your hands in front; or raise one hand off the ground at a time to brush your nose, then lower to continue the Muaythai push-up and spring back up to the preparation position.

Handstand Posture

ท่าหกสูง

Tha = Posture; ***Hok Sung*** = Handstand

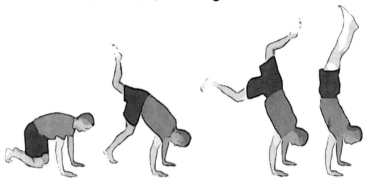

Preparation: Kneel and place your hands underneath your shoulders with your fingers spread wide, arms straight.

Movement: Raise one leg up together with your hips and continue to gently swing your leg and hips up. Your other leg will follow and once you have found your balance hold the position. Both arms must remain straight throughout.

It is recommended that you start training nearby a wall, which acts as a safety net and allows you to build up your confidence. The wall needs to be about the distance of six fists away from your hands. Initially, practise to just swing your leg up until you get the feel for the right amount of effort required and are able to support your own body weight. Only progress when ready. If you feel yourself losing your balance, immediately drop one of your feet back down.

Focus: Remain positive.

Active Form: Maintain the posture.

Inhale: Swing one leg up.   **Exhale:** To return.

Inhale and Exhale: Natural breath movement as you maintain posture.

Channel and Intensify Life Force: Let your energy rise upwards, out through your toes and high up into the sky.

Muscular Area: Spine / Core-abs and back / Upper back / Shoulders / Arms / Wrists / Hands.

Benefit: Balance / Focus / Positive thinking / Confidence / Coordination / Circulation / Flow of blood to brain / Reverses effect of gravity / Sensory abilities / Eye focus with soft gaze / Unique perspective when upside down.

Self-Defence: Preparation for an advanced technique called the Cartwheel Kick / An excellent way to overcome fear / Balance in all defence and attack techniques.

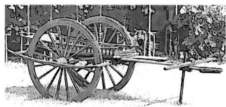

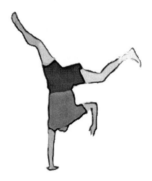

Interest: There are many Muay techniques hidden within traditional Thai dance. Being able to balance on your hands forms one of the primary exercises of dance and enables students to literally walk on their hands and do somersaults. It is a beautiful display of freedom of movement.

The posture is also known as Downward Facing Tree.

Variation: You can also try it with your legs out wide.

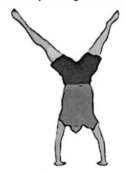

Monkey Posture

ท่าลิง

Tha = Posture; *Ling* = Monkey

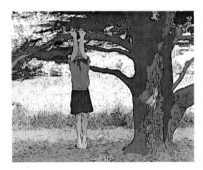 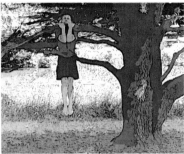

Preparation: Grip the branch or bar with your palms facing you, body extended.

Movement: Bend your arms to raise your head above your monkey grip. Keep your elbows together.

Focus: Maintain stillness in the rest of your body.

Active Form: Continuous flow.

Passive Form: Hold the preparation position.

Inhale: As you lift up.

Exhale: As you lower.

Inhale and Exhale: Natural breath movement as you hold the positions.

Channel and Intensify Life Force: Visualize a giant pulling you up and only contract the muscles needed.

Purpose:
Muscular Area: Core / Back / Back of shoulders / Front of arms / Hands.
Benefit: Releases the spine from the negative effects of gravity / Increases metabolic rate / Bone density.
Self-Defence: Develops good form and power for an inside grapple position. By squeezing your elbows in, it forms a vice-like clamp that strangles your opponent slightly and gives you the advantage of the higher ground. It gives you the best position to launch knee strikes / Grip in locks and breaks.

Interest: The Hanuman Langur is named after Hanuman (Monkey God). The Langur is fast and agile like the wind and has strength through a vast range of motion. Other qualities include balance and courage. All this is gained through time spent hanging in the trees.

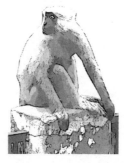

Interest: The modern Thai military do many pull-ups. If you can pull up 100% of your body weight, you may have all the strength you need.

Variation: Simply hang straight to decompress your spine.

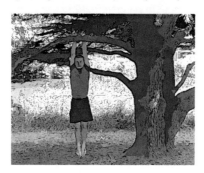

Achieving Extraordinary Energy and Power

Just using technique is not enough to succeed in Muay. The following methods will give you the extra energy and power you need to be a successful Muay warrior.

You cannot learn these methods by just seeing or reading about them because they are quite hidden and very difficult to see. Therefore, it is essential to tune into your senses to feel them, and when you do, it can feel like magic. You will need to feel these methods to gain a deeper understanding and greater awareness of them. Practise them and achieve a new form of power and energy.

If you combine the methods you will sense extraordinary energy and power.

Creating a Firm Foundation

It is essential to master the methods in this chapter so that you gain a firm foundation. This will enable you to positively advance and progress. Once you have a strong foundation, everything flows from it easily and more powerfully.

Many of the ways can be practised in training and in everyday life.

Life Force
(Phalang Khong Chiwit)

Thai people call life force (vital energy) *Phalang Khong Chiwit.*

Life force is inside us and all around us. We absorb it through air (breath), sunlight, the earth, food and water. Life force is everywhere. It binds us all together. In Muay, you learn to connect with the life force, cultivate it and use it wisely.

Thai people believe that it flows through about 72,000 channels in the body called *Sen* lines. All the *Sen* lines begin at the navel. If the *Sen* lines become blocked it can lead to poor health. Practising Muay postures encourages energy to flow freely along these *Sen* lines resulting in good health, vitality and power.

This ancient way of training the life force has almost been lost due to modern Muay Thai, but it has remained an important part of Thai Massage and Thai Yoga (The Hermit's Body Twist. Rusie Dotton).

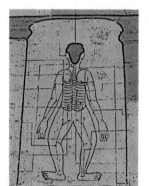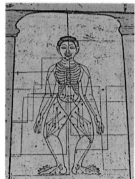

Sen lines

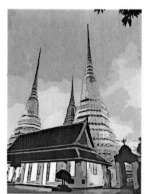

Medicine Pavilion, Wat Pho, Bangkok.

Thai people also use the synonyms จี *chi (qi)* or ปราณ ลม *pran lom (prana)* when referring to life force.

Feel it- Firstly, move your fingertips in and out without touching your opponent's arm. Be mindful, relax and take full natural breaths. Secondly, move your fingertips up and down their arm, fingertips close but not touching. You may find it helpful and more powerful to visualize life force flowing between your fingertips. Take it in turns.

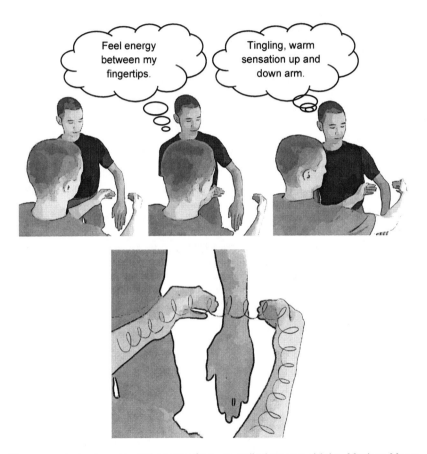

Many people try to gain vital energy from so-called energy drinks. Modern Muay Thai even heavily promotes them. People will go to extremes to search for energy, including climbing great mountains. The best way to get energy is simply to conserve it and stop wasting it. Relax to absorb it and build it up.

Warning- Excess sugar intake will zap your energy, suppress your immune system and cause muscles to lose their elasticity.

Channel and Intensify Life Force

This is the way you can train each Muay posture to come alive, increase intensity and continually progress without limitations. It creates lines of life force, channels vital energy and intensifies the flow through the *sen* lines. It is also a great way to discover through practice, a magical kind of power.

Expressing your energy in the following ways has many benefits. It will help you to lengthen, expand, widen and open your joints. It also saves energy and creates energy, increasing power. Having faith and mastering it become powerful allies and will give you a huge advantage over the average person.

Imagine vital energy flowing through lines within your body and beyond into the earth or air. To intensify energy you can visualize more current flowing through the lines. You must maintain softness in the body by only using the muscles you need, and so balancing the active with the passive.

Become aware of the dynamic opposition. This is when one part of your body moves in one direction, whilst the opposite part moves in the opposite direction. Visualize life force flowing through lines in the body and beyond. The source of the life force that flows through the lines is always from the centre, which opens up as opposite parts of the body move in opposite directions.

Feel it- Firstly, kneel in front of your partner and lift your arms so they are level with your shoulders. Tense your whole body. Get your partner to push down on to your arms. Secondly, visualize a line of life force flowing through your arms and continuing beyond. Tune into your body and feel the difference.

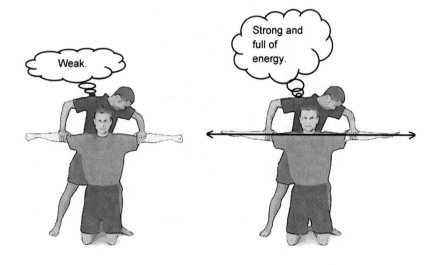

For variation, you can also try the following, which will give the same effect. Visualize pressing against two rocks at the end of each energy line. As you get more efficient and you want to boost the flow of energy, you can increase the press to 25 per cent of your strength, then to 50 per cent, up to 100 per cent. Remember to maintain softness and also visualize the perfect posture.

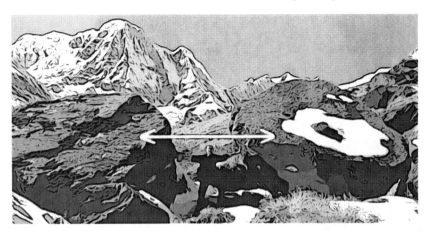

Feel it- Firstly, punch a pad with a straight punch. Secondly, start to rotate your arm slowly, then quickly about ten times and release a straight punch to the pad. The rotations build up vital energy in your hand. Apply caution by using hand wraps. For added protection you may need to double wrap your wrist.

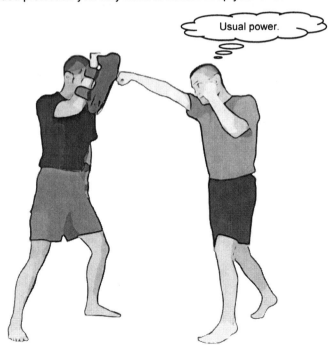

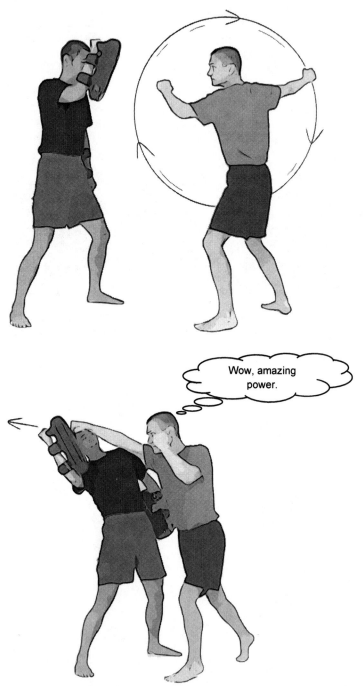

This is an exercise in itself, without hitting a pad. It is an excellent way of releasing tension in the shoulders and upper torso.

Crucial Life Force Channel

The *Sen* line called *Sen Sumana* is one of the most important life force channels in the body. Good spine posture is essential because *Sen Sumana* is located along the midline of the body. A natural lengthening of the spine in all the postures enables life force, including spiritual energy, to flow well. Good posture also prevents tension and gives the impression of confidence.

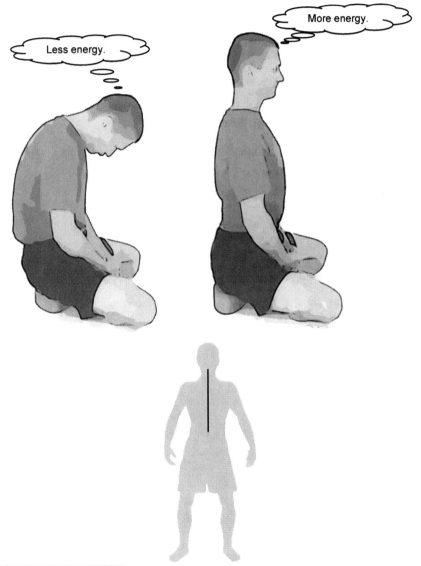

Integration Practice- Throughout your day become aware of your posture and correct it if necessary.

Breath of Life –
Natural Breath Movement
(Lom Haichai)

The most important and easiest way we absorb and create life force (vital energy) is through the air that we breathe. No breath, no life. Thai people call this *Lom Haichai* meaning breath of life. It is the way of the natural breath movement. When we are young we all breathe naturally but as we get older, with all the stresses and strains of life, some of us lose this natural ability.

The practice of the natural breath in Muay allows you to distribute and store more life force. This has the effect of purifying the *Sen* energy lines and increasing the flow of vital energy, making you powerful. The breath of life also connects your body to the mind. Calm breath, calm mind.

Feel it- Place your fingertips together on your belly. Breathe from your belly.

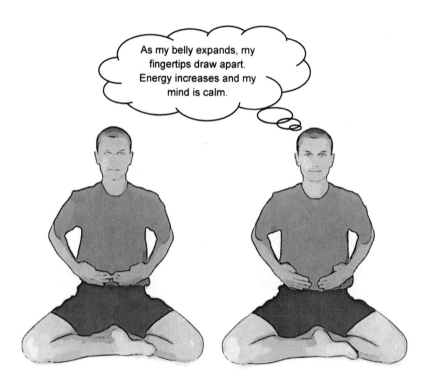

As my belly expands, my fingertips draw apart. Energy increases and my mind is calm.

Nine Qualities of the Natural Breath Movement

- Slow (unhurried)
- Fine (smooth)
- Quiet
- Long (steady stream of air)
- Complete (full, deep breath using whole lung capacity, breathing from the belly)
- Even (balanced inhale and exhale, through both nostrils, mouth closed)
- Tranquil (peaceful with no disturbance, mind focused on present experience, free of thoughts and worries)
- Synchronized (in harmony with movement)
- Relaxed (no tension, if the breath is not relaxed the body cannot relax)

Note: As you exhale, this is the opportunity to soften and let go. Take advantage of this by deepening the posture as you breathe out.

Breath cultivates patience as well as energy.

Warning- Do not try and control your breath, this only leads to tension.

When you breathe, imagine absorbing life force rather than just air.

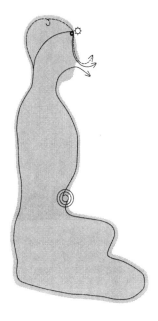

Understanding the Mind

To understand how the mind works take a look up at the blue sky and see the similarities with your mind.

The blue sky, like your mind (calm and clear, no thoughts)

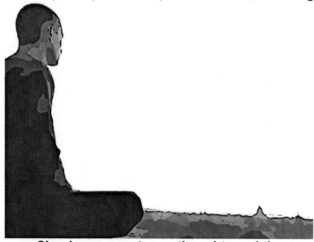

Clouds represent your thoughts and the colour of the clouds, your emotions (nothing but thoughts)

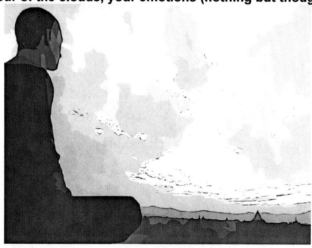

Note how the clouds come and go and that the blue sky is always there.

Non-stop thoughts (clouds) prevent us from observing the mind (calm and clear blue sky).

The blue sky represents mindfulness (awareness and being present)

In Muay we aim to discover the blue sky and search for happiness and peace from within, rather than from the outside.

Challenge- Try and locate you emotions.

After some time you may find that they are hard to find. Like clouds, emotions and thoughts have no substance to them. Yet without training they can have an extremely negative effect on us.

The way we respond to thoughts and emotions can give us problems. Thoughts and emotions are not problems. When we train in mindfulness, they lose their power over us.

Mindfulness (Khwam Mi Sati)

Moment to moment awareness enables you to train and defend in battle skilfully to achieve your aims. Mindfulness makes it possible to deal with situations and respond wisely. It will enable you to be clear and focused without distraction.

Mindfulness is extremely powerful. It gives you the energy, softness and balance that you need in training and in battle.

Warning- A mind that is not calm is unaware and distracted. With non-stop thoughts and emotions that are high or low, it only allows your inner enemies (anger, fear, impatience, ego, desires and so on) to harm you, or you become at their mercy.

A mind that is constantly in the future or the past, exhausts life force.

To calm the mind, you must practise focusing and quietening the mind. Clarity and awareness will then arise.

To be present, you must practise being in the here and now. Clarity and awareness will then arise.

Mindfulness　　　　**Mind full**

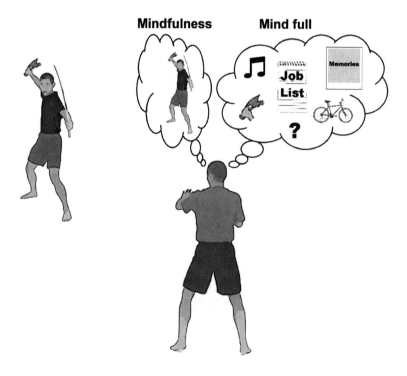

Meditation

You need to practise mindfulness (awareness and being present) in the same way as you need to practise physical movements and the way to do it is through daily meditation. This will help you to integrate mindfulness into everyday life. It will enable you to regain control of your mind and body.

Ultimately, it can help you to achieve the main aim of Muay - Oneness.

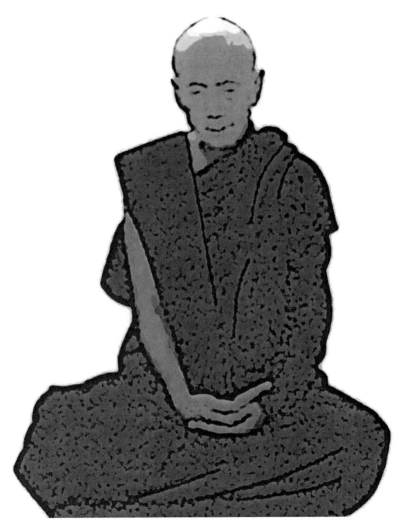

The majority of people in Thailand are Buddhist and a large percentage of Thai males become monks during some part of their lives. Meditation is an integral part of Buddhist practice and there are many techniques. The following gives you a simple guide on how to practise meditation.

Preparation for Meditation and How to Practise:
1. Choose a place and time that is peaceful and free from distractions.
2. To help connect with nature, face east or north and meditate at dawn or dusk.
3. Sit in the meditation posture. This will cultivate energy, stillness and balance. Ensure that you are in a firm position and relaxed throughout.
Eyes closed.
Chin slightly down.
Upright posture with a natural curve in spine.
Right hand resting on top of left. Tips of your thumbs touching.
Knees and buttocks connect to the earth and form a triangle circuit of life force.
4. Instruct your mind to be calm and present.
5. Breathe calmly with full natural breathes.
6. Rest your mind on a focal point, for example, the *unalom* (third eye).
7. Do not battle with restlessness of the mind. If thoughts arise, treat them like clouds on a windy day, just let them come and go.
8. When we concentrate there is firm control over the mind. We start to meditate when this control is no longer needed.
9. With practice you will start to observe your actions, thoughts and emotions. Avoid identifying with them and just witness them. Distance yourself from them.

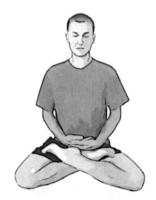

Applying Mindfulness
Muay warriors aim to practise mindfulness in everything they do.

In Muay training, you first become more mindful of the physical movement, then as you progress you also tune into the energetic body, the movement of breath and life force.

Integration Practice- Begin to add mindfulness into your everyday life by selecting at least one activity per day to practise moment to moment awareness. Soon you will be able to apply mindfulness to more and more things that you do in your life.

Awareness of Weaknesses

To improve you must first become aware of your weaknesses. The spirit and courage of the Muay warrior is needed to accept and then deal with the weaknesses. You may need to battle with desire as it may be tempting to only focus on your strengths because it feels uplifting and motivating. It is also through learning about and focusing on your weaknesses that will create balance and allow you to progress.

Be aware of weaknesses of the body and mind. The real challenge comes when you deal with weaknesses of the mind (mental and emotional). They are harder to deal with than the physical because they are difficult to observe and you identify with them more. You have to be free of resistance and defensiveness when dealing with them.

Many weaknesses often remain hidden or come to our attention too late when we suffer poor health. When you start to train in awareness you may start to notice lots of weaknesses and it may feel like you are not progressing. Maintain the spirit of the Muay warrior and be armed with positivity, courage, faith and confidence. Keep practising and do not get disheartened.

Awareness Friend

A mirror can be used occasionally as it is an excellent awareness friend. It will give you instant and honest visual feedback on your physical strengths and weaknesses and therefore the knowledge required to improve.

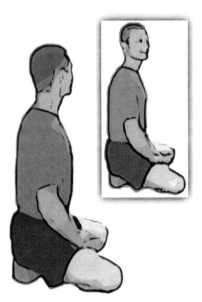

The Edge (Awareness Zone)

This is the place where you feel a comfortable stretch in the posture. The edge is the point of balance between doing too much or too little.

It is important to find the edge because it is where you will be safe, achieve results and gather wisdom about yourself.

You can train the edge when using the passive form of the posture. Be patient and wait until you feel relaxed at the edge, then deepen the posture with subtle movements. As you further the edge, your flexibility and strength will increase.

In the section Essentials of Muay Training (p.155), it describes the ways that will help you to train and improve the edge, including the use of the breath, energy lines and awareness. Being skilful in the postures of Muay is about being able to train the edges well, so you can be very skilful at Muay without being super supple.

Remember to use the out breath to help you to go further and deeper into the posture.

Once you have achieved a greater range than before, ensure to hold the posture for a least one natural breath movement.

Do not battle with yourself, use oneness and your energy wisely. Stretch, do not stress.

Positive Thinking (Kan Mong Lok Nai Ngae Di)

Being positive and confident is extremely powerful. It not only feels better but is essential for success in all that you do. An opponent can often sense it if you have it and that alone may deter them.

Tip- You can practise with daily positive affirmations.

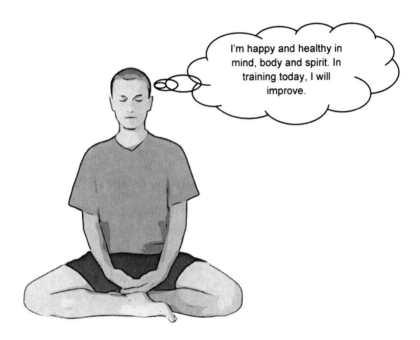

I'm happy and healthy in mind, body and spirit. In training today, I will improve.

Note- Positivity attracts positivity, for example, a smile is usually returned with a smile.

Turn a negative situation into a positive one. For example, if someone throws you a punch, they have also given away some of their balance to you and created gaps which you can take advantage of. In another instance, if someone throws bananas at you, create a banana stall and sell them. Always be armed with a sense of humour!

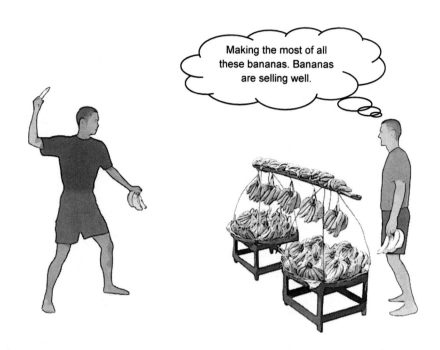

Integration Practice- Everyday have a go at making a mental list of nine positive things. These could include things that you are grateful for and that are in the present moment. The last few can be a real challenge and that is when your awareness will deepen.

Balance (Sama Dun)

Wholeness and good health arises when all is balanced.

Every quality of Muay requires balance.

Once balance is attained, excellent performance in Muay will follow and also fast recovery.

Uniting and Balancing the Opposites

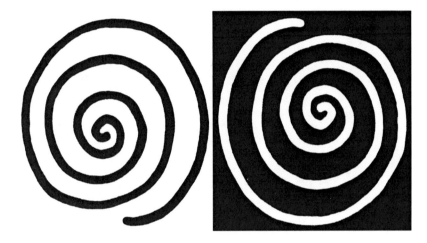

Opposites exist together and complement each other.

Life force (vital energy) arises from the interaction of opposites.

Muay postures help you to achieve balance between the opposite forces of nature. Begin by becoming aware of the imbalance, this can be tough because they may feel normal to you. To gain balance you may need to apply the opposite energy. Too much or too little of either can result in poor health. Aim for the middle way.

Feel it- Select a target and a few objects to throw at it. The example uses a Thai pad and boxing wraps. Stand a few meters away. If you throw too high and miss, do the opposite by aiming too low on the next throw. If you throw too far to one side, next aim too far the opposite side of the target.

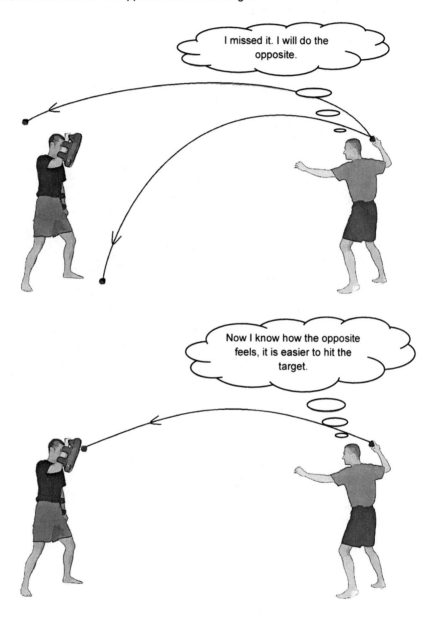

Note- Doing the opposite may feel weird or uncomfortable but it will help you to find balance or the middle way.

If one aspect of the duality is out of balance, it may have an effect on any other aspect, for example, if the mind is unbalanced, the body will be imbalanced.

Feel it- When you feel calm, hold a position that requires balance. Then try to hold the same position, for example, when you feel angry or upset. Notice and feel the difference.

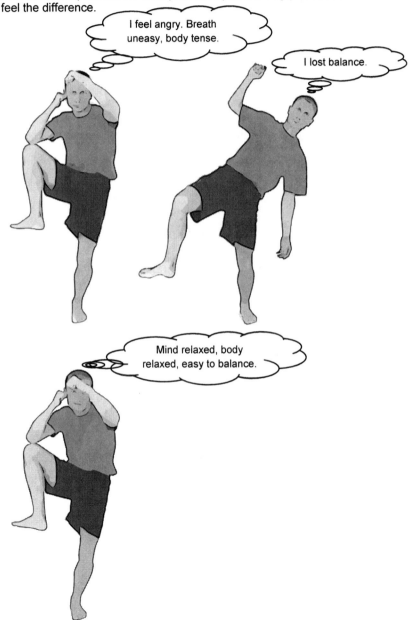

Note- To challenge your balance even more, practise with your eyes shut.

Tip- To deal with emotional imbalances you must first become aware of them. Then consciously start to take full natural breaths and relax your body. When emotions are out of balance, the breath becomes uneasy and the body tenses up.

Three Unwholesome Roots (Akusonlamun Sam)

The toughest battle in life is often with inner enemies known as the Three Unwholesome Roots. They cause lack of mindfulness, tension, imbalance, poor breathing, negative thinking and suffering to the mind and body.

Hate (Anger, Envy)
Greed (Desire, Attachment)
Delusion (Bewilderment, Ignorance)

Three Wholesome Roots (Kusonlamun Sam)

Once you practise becoming aware of the unwholesome roots you can start to defend yourself with their opposites, known as the Three Wholesome Roots. Aim to cultivate and create good habits of them.

Non-Hatred (Love, Kindness, Patience, Calmness, Compassion)
Non-Greed (Generosity, Contentment, Detachment)
Non-Delusion (Wisdom, Understanding, Truth)

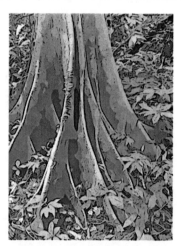

Wholesome roots can triumph over unwholesome roots.

The Unity of Dualities Specific to Muay

Sun	Moon
Fire	Water
Air	Earth
Rama (Hero King)	Tosakanth (Demon King)
Right Side	Left Side
Positive	Negative
Hot	Cold
Sun Breath (Right Nostril)	Moon Breath (Left Nostril)
Male Triangle Stance	Female Triangle Stance
Active Form	Passive Form
Effort	Release
In Motion (Angry Tiger)	In Rest (Hibernating Naga)
Exhale	Inhale
Attack	Defence
Outside	Inside
Upward	Downward
Aggressive	Calm
Outward Energy	Inward Energy
Courage	Fear
Patience	Impatience
Firm	Yielding
Upper	Lower
Heavens	Underworld

An old Thai proverb about Muay warriors is "fierce as a lion, gentle as a lamb".

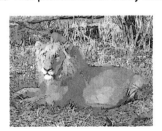 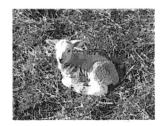

In Thai culture, the story of Garuda and Naga is an excellent representation of these dualities. They are commonly associated with each other and recognized by the opposite characteristics they symbolize. Their opposing qualities create balance and equilibrium.

Garuda is a mighty bird who is king of the birds. He is half man, half bird. Naga is a dragon-like serpent snake. They are in constant battle with each other. The feud started when their mothers married the same powerful sage.

The pair form the emblem for King Rama II.

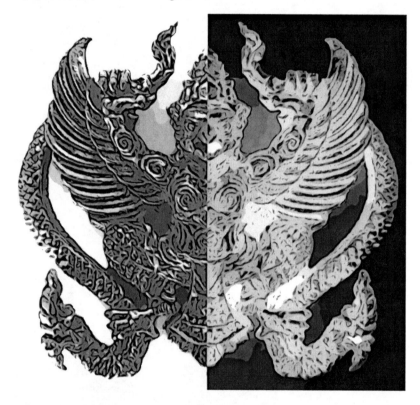

Garuda represents the light forces of nature, the heavens, sun, fire and air.

Naga represents the dark forces of nature, the underworld, moon, water and earth.

Balancing the Principles

A balanced lifestyle and creating good habits are necessary to form a strong overall foundation and achieve excellence.

Body Training
Mind Training
Relaxing (Softness)
Breathing (Life Force)
Healthy Eating

The majority of people know what a healthy lifestyle is and what good habits are. The difficulty is in adopting them.

You can create a positive habit or lose a negative habit instantly. After about 30 days of change you will be winning the battle. It is the good habits that will enable you to be constant in your training. You may have more success changing only one bad habit at a time.

Balancing the Elements

Muay helps you to achieve harmony between all the elements. It balances, purifies and opens up powers of each element to achieve good health.

Thai people believe that there are four elements *(that)* ธาตุ.

Earth (*Din*) ดิน
Water (*Nam*) น้ำ
Fire (*Fai*) ไฟ
Air/Wind (*Lom*) ลม

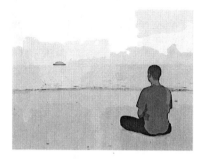

Each element is associated to specific *Sen* lines, parts of the body and states of the mind.

Qualities associated with each element		
Element	**Body**	**Mind**
Earth	Solid grounding / central fulcrum that other elements move round / good posture	Confidence
Water	Flowing / yielding / elusive / softness (non-resistance) / repetition / synchronization of the breath and movement	Adaptable, flexible and reflective
Fire	Explosive power / speed / action / change / body locks	Motivated and passionate
Air	Freedom to move / growth / breath	Open minded

All qualities are maintained even under stress.

Interest: The irrepressible powers and energy of the four elements are demonstrated in hurricanes, volcanoes, earthquakes and tidal waves.

Connecting to the Earth

Achieve balance and increase life force in the following ways:
- Distribute your body weight evenly.
- Maintain a calm mind.
- Soften whole body to stay rooted to the earth (p.139).
- Keep your knee and elbow joints soft so they are not locked out.
- Spread your toes wide in standing postures.
- Create a wide stance when possible.
- Awareness and usage of your centre of gravity (p.134).

An ideal time to practise these is whilst training in the Muay postures.

Feel it- By simply putting your feet together and moving your upper body and upper limbs you become extremely unstable. Never give your balance away like this.

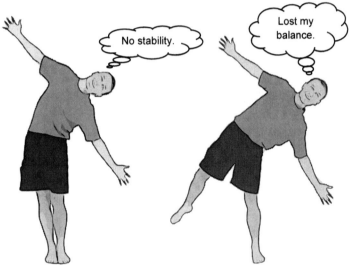

Integration Practice- Get into a good habit by creating an everyday stance, standing with your knees soft and your feet shoulder width apart. Body weight is evenly spread out over the soles of your feet.

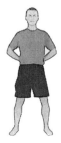

Note- A Muay warrior rarely stands with their feet together and legs locked out. The wide stance feels more comfortable, stable and balanced and improves the flow of energy.

Centring

Having a wide stance gives you firm support for your centre of gravity and allows your centre greater movement. The lower your centre of gravity is, the better your balance will be.

Your centre of gravity is located just below your belly button, in the centre of your body.

If you can feel for your opponent's centre of gravity you can easily off-balance them.

All of the postures in Muay can give you the ability to be aware and utilize the muscles around your centre. By improving these powerhouse muscles you will gain fluidity, greater power and balance. An armour of muscle will also protect your vital organs.

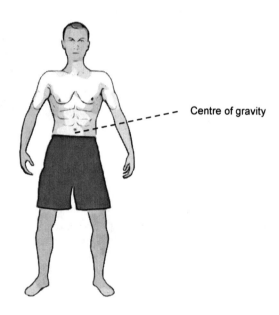

Centre of gravity

Relax (Kan Phon Khlai)

This is power free from tension.

The rewards of becoming soft and relaxed include:
- Deeper natural breath movement.
- Absorbing and filling up with vital energy from the elements.
- Cultivating vital energy which also flows more freely.
- Conserving energy, focusing it for where or when you need it.
- Reinvigorates.
- Speedy recovery.
- Allowing muscles to stretch.
- Absorbing effects of posture.
- Letting go of tension and unwanted toxins in the body.
- Increases speed.
- Tune into senses.
- Gain balance.

How- Mindfulness, breathing and letting go will allow your mind and body to relax.

Tip- Frequently scanning the body can help you to become aware of tension.

You may need to consciously tense up to help you become aware of tension before you can let it go. A simple technique you can practise throughout the day is to tense, shake, breathe and relax.

Tip- Cultivating contentment in lifestyle and situations will also keep you relaxed. Desires and attachments may lead to fear, frustration and tension. Search for contentment on the inside rather than from the outside.

Effort and Release Pattern

You can relax by releasing between the postures. This will enable you to practise the opposites, effort / release.

This pattern can also be practised when doing combinations on the Thai pads. Going from steady (not stopping) to fully committed.

During stressful situations, our bodies react by tensing up and releasing chemicals such as adrenaline to help us through these troubled times. Even if you felt you were successful in dealing with the stressful situation, your problem may continue because tension and chemicals remain stored within you, which if is persistent, can result in disease, illness and injury. Training in effort / release will avoid this happening and keep your mind and body in balance.

Remember to also relax throughout the postures using only the muscles that you need.

Softness

Use your awareness to release tension and allow the body soften. You will save energy and focus it for where or when you need it with increased speed. Speed is power. Stay relaxed but do not become like a soft noodle.

Feel & Integrate it- With everything you do, do it with minimum effort. If you continue to do this you will start to feel the difference in yourself. The example below illustrates the difference between tension and relaxation in doing something so simple such as talking on the phone.

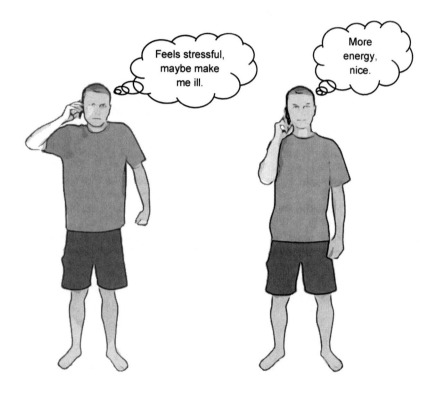

Note- Softness is a characteristic that is very much apparent in Thai warriors. This quality is cultivated through their way of life and mastered in training. This softness enables suppleness and strength which is seen in their fighting style and is a pleasure to watch.

Important Note- You can stretch muscles that are soft (contraction free). You cannot stretch muscles that are tense.

It is amazing how flexible you can become if you simply stay relaxed throughout the day.

Important Choice- Do you want to feel alive, be flexible and flowing with energy like the branch of a tree? Or would you rather be a stick that is stiff, resistant, with no life force in it and so easily breaks? It is up to you!

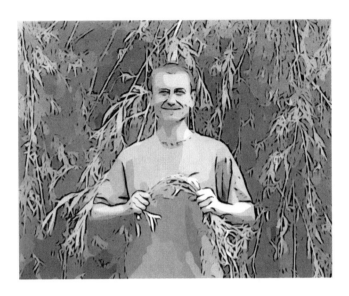

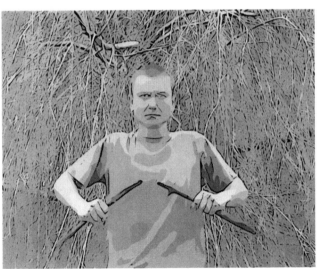

Sense of Touch

Softness will also help you to tune into your senses. With a better sense of touch, you will increase your awareness.

Feel it- Pick up an object when you are totally tense and then again when you are totally relaxed. Feel the difference.

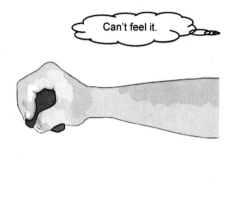

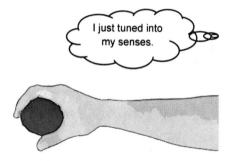

Your weapon against tension is simply to soften and relax the body.

With everything you do, do it with minimum effort.

Remain positive as it will help keep you relaxed and avoid trying as this leads to tension.

Sinking

Become rooted to the earth. This enables you to focus your life force to where it is required and draw vital energy from the earth.

In battle it will assist you in taking an opponent down or make it extremely difficult for your opponent to take you down. The way to achieve this is by softening your whole body so that it becomes heavy and relaxed. A full natural breath and a calm mind is also necessary.

Feel it- Ask someone (who is able) to lift you, first when you are tense and then when you are relaxed and see if you can notice the difference.

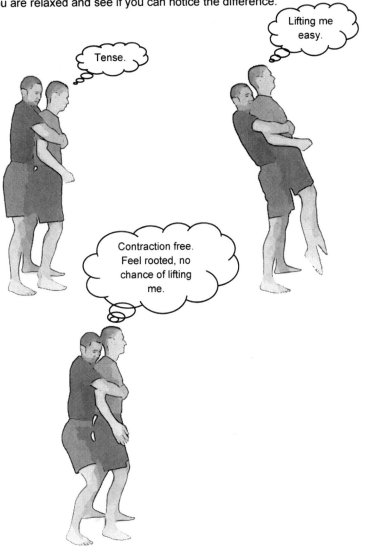

Aim to be Childlike

In Muay we aim to return to our natural form, to become as flexible, mindful, relaxed and open minded as when we were young.

Muay can rejuvenate.

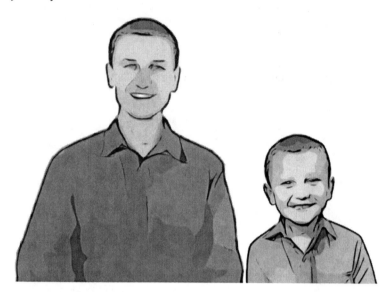

Freshness

Every battle is different and life is continually changing. So the way of the Muay warrior is to always keep an open mind and approach everything you do with freshness and a feeling of newness.

Integration Practice- Everyday try something new or do something slightly different without any expectations. This will help you to practise mindfulness and has the effect of opening your mind and changing your perspective. It may even help you become aware of negative habits.

The Routines

This section has a few routines that you can use as a quick reference guide. Each routine has a main focus and for a complete routine you need to do them all. They have been developed to be balanced and whole. All parts of the body are trained equally. The postures in each routine include inversions, forward bends, back bends, twists and balances. The postures complement and augment each other. Feel free to use other suitable postures in the book as alternatives.

Our bodies and weaknesses are all different so it can be more beneficial for you to design your own routine. Ensure that it is balanced or aims to make you balanced. Always counterbalance a forward bend with a back bend. A posture that compresses must be followed with one that extends. Train your lower, core, upper and both sides of the body equally. Twists can be refreshing after forward and back bends.

It is important to warm up before you begin the sequence of postures. There is a warm up routine included as a suggestion. One of the best ways to warm up if you know how to, is to do a Muay dance.

Traditionally Thai people start from low to high because it counters the effects of gravity and life force purifies as it rises. Postures that emphasize the lower part of the body are done first, then the mid (core) part of the body and finally, the upper part.

Avoid doing too many standing postures. This can lead to aggression.

Initially, do one set of about 30 seconds until you have learnt how to do the posture and then build up to at least three sets of a minute.

Train on alternating days to allow your body the rest it needs and to adapt to becoming stronger and more flexible.

With the strength training, the slower you go the harder you will train. Generally, one complete movement of the posture is synchronised with a complete natural breath movement. The breath will help to guide your pace.

Requirements For Progression In Strength	
Frequency	3 times per week
Intensity	3 sets on each area (4 sets max) Going slower increases intensity
Time	30 - 90 seconds each or 3 - 6 natural breath movements
Type	Active form

Requirements For Progression In Flexibility	
Frequency	3 times per week
Intensity	3 sets on each area (4 sets max) Train the edge (awareness zone)
Time	30 - 90 seconds each or 3 - 6 natural breath movements
Type	Passive form

Cardiovascular and technique training is also a major part of Muay including training with Thai pads, punch bags, running and so on. It is recommended that you do at least 20 minutes of cardiovascular training three times a week.

Daily warm ups, cat stretches and meditation are also important to include in the complete routine.

Warm Up Routine

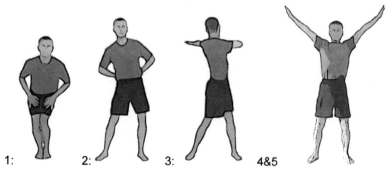

1:    2:   3:   4&5

1: Shortened Body Posture, p.21
2: Stir the Energy Posture, p.22
3: Charging Army Posture, p.23
4: Elephant Destroying the Holding Pen, p.26
5: Tiger Destroying the Hunter's Tree Hide, p.28

Strength Routine

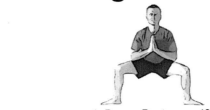

1: Dance Posture, p.43

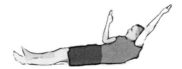

2: Hermit Crushes Medicine Posture, p.68

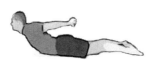

3: Arrow Posture, p.72

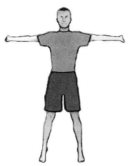

4: Breath Moving Posture, p.85

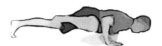

5: Muaythai Push-up and Knee Block, p.97

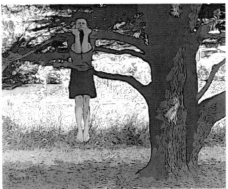

6: Monkey Posture, p.105

Flexibility Routine

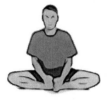

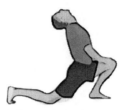

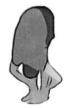

1: Salute Earth Posture, p.57

2: Salute Star Posture, p.49

3: Mountain Embracing Posture, p.51

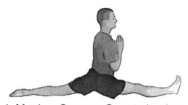

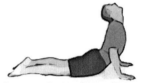

4: Monkey Crosses Over to Lanka, p.53

5: Serpent Snake with a Crystal in its Mouth Posture, p.74

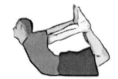

6: Bow Posture, p.73

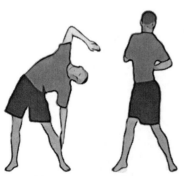

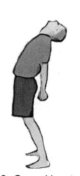

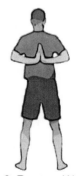

7: Mountain Hiding Posture, p.80

8: Open Heart Posture, p.89

9: Reverse Wai Posture, p.90

144

Life Force and Internal Power Routine

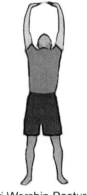
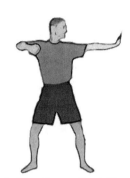

1: Tri Worship Posture, p.58

2: King Draws Back Bow and Arrow Posture, p.86

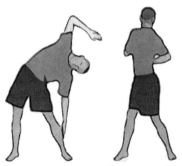

3: Mountain Hiding Posture, p.80

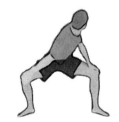
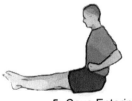

4: Giant Turns Posture, p.78

5: Cave Entering Posture, p.55

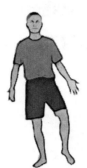
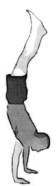

6: Ward off Illness Posture
(Tense, Shake, Breathe),
p.32

7: Handstand Posture,
p.103

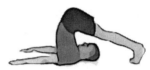

8: God of Air / Wind Clears and Brightens Posture,
p.66

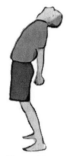
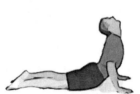
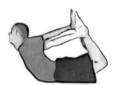

9: Open Heart
Posture,
p.89

10: Serpent Snake with a
Crystal in its Mouth Posture,
p.74

11: Bow Posture,
p.73

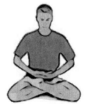

12. Meditation Posture,
p.34

Train in Harmony with Nature

Traditionally, all training was done outdoors to achieve optimum health, allowing the warrior to connect with the vital energy within them and the fresh vital energy around them. The modern Muay warrior often adapts the training with Thai pads and punch bags and so on. This is okay but you should only utilize what you need. It is amazing what you can achieve without all the fancy gear.

Nature is one of the greatest teachers. Use your awareness to learn from it.

Warning- The egotist becomes stiff, inflexible and weak if they do not connect with their surroundings.

Nature's Gym

Lines in the dirt and coconut shells for footwork practice.

Strike hanging limes for practising defence as they swing.

Water splashed in eyes by striking down on the surface for eyesight focus.

Kick banana plants, aim to chop it down and to keep it up, to condition the shins.

Strike leaves to practise speed and distance precision.

Downward elbow strikes on to coconuts to condition the elbows.

Climb trees to improve grappling.

Running in deep water and air boxing (shadow boxing) for enhancing the cardiovascular system.

Train footwork in slippery mud to become more proficient.

Push kicks to tree trunks to toughen up soles of feet. Walking barefoot is also a great way to harden the soles of the feet, essential for preventing blisters when pivoting feet on techniques.

Sitting on a tree trunk whilst a partner launches strikes to practise defence.

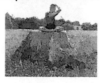

Please note that this chapter is intended to give you an understanding of how the ancient Thai warrior connected with energy around them, rather than part of a training routine.

The Three Part Strategy

It is essential to master a simple strategy to become a winner without fighting. It is more likely that it will be a novice Muay warrior that needs to fight. Rarely will you see a master fight and only in defence of themselves or others.

A simple order of strategy to apply before you attack is:

1st Avoidance

Be aware of the threat and quietly walk or run away from the situation.

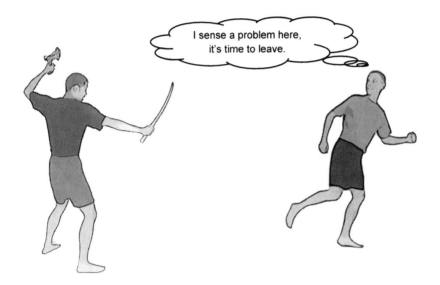

> I sense a problem here, it's time to leave.

If the potential for danger is in your way, then the simplest thing to do is move out of the way. Do not resist.

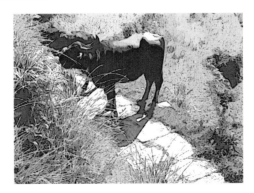

2ⁿᵈ Diplomacy

In Thailand the *wai* (respectful greeting) is like the handshake. It has the same effect of achieving a peaceful resolution, whilst also putting you in a better guard position. It also gives you time to talk calmly and politely to resolve any problems.

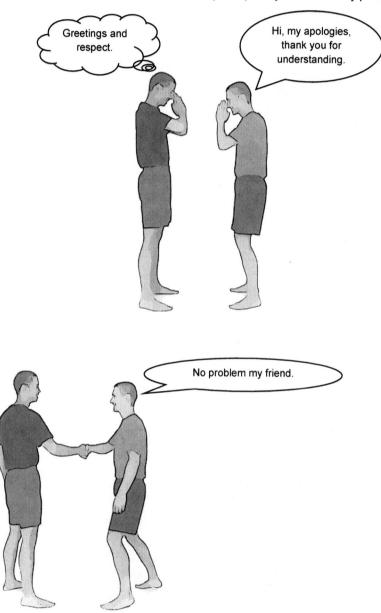

3rd Warning

Give a confident and non-aggressive verbal warning. You must maintain and guard your distance even if all seems fine. Show confidence by avoiding stepping back. If you cannot maintain your distance, or you need to move back more than twice, you are in danger and it is time to attack.

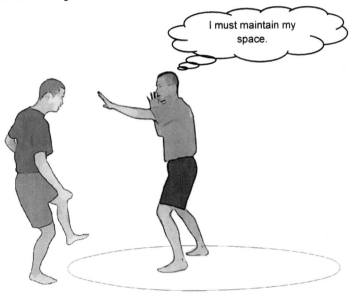

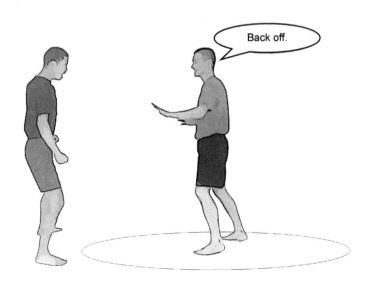

The Three Thai Ways

Ideally, the best strategy is a combination of the Three Part Strategy along with the following Three Thai Ways.

All three of these Thai ways are common qualities of the people of Thailand. They are useful to practise and learn when doing Thai martial arts because they provide an excellent way to maintain peace, helping to avoid trouble and deal with problems. The Thai ways can also help you achieve happiness, fulfillment and longevity.

Note-
In the true spirit of these ways, they should be done with a smile.

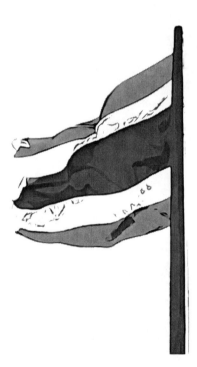

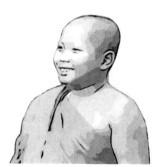

1st Chai Yen

Chai Yen is translated as cool heart. Keep a cool heart at all times.

How-
If a problem or situation arises you must respond by being patient, relaxed and calm. Even if you do not really feel like this, you must restrain yourself and not show it. For example, respond with a smile even if you feel angry. Being angry has no value in Muay and can be harmful if it builds up.

2nd Kreng Chai

The definition of *Kreng Chai* is to be understanding, considerate and respectful of another person.

How-
Simply become aware of someone else's feelings and desires. This is important, especially when people deserve it or need it when there is a problem. A sign of a good Muay warrior is one that can show empathy and compassion.

You should always practise *Kreng Chai* when training with a partner.

3rd Mai Pen Rai

Mai pen rai means nevermind, it does not matter.

How-
Do not make a big deal of situations or problems. This is sometimes not easy but you have to accept the situation or problem and learn to let things go.

A wise old master was asked to reveal his secret for long life. He replied by saying "I just don't make a big deal out of things." Principally, this has helped him to stay healthy and live longer but also benefits others by making those around him feel a lot better too.

Tip-
You can only control yourself. You cannot control your opponent.

A way to learn to control yourself when dealing with stressful situations or problems is to follow these three steps:
1st Accept it.
2nd Be aware of your aims, what do you want out of it?
3rd Apply what you need to do to achieve your aims.

Tough Times

A storm can represent challenging or stressful times.
Shelter under the following and know that storms, like tough times, do not last.
Remember there is always a blue sky above the storm.

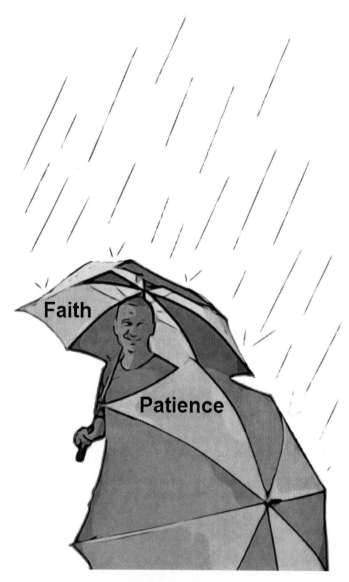

Shine in a storm. Practising Muay through tough times may feel extremely challenging and you may feel least like doing it, but it will be when you need it the most. It too can give you shelter from a long storm as well as a feeling of continuity. Storms can make you stronger.

The spirals on Hanuman's arm symbolizes the journey of life, growth and change. It also symbolizes the movement of energy. `- - - - -`

Training Session Essentials

The following essentials act as a quick reminder of what you need to apply once you have learnt good technique. Technique alone is not enough. In each training session, get in the habit of applying and combining the following powers:

Life-Force (Phalang Khong Chiwit)
Connect with the energy around you. Create a dynamic opposition. Visualize the flow of energy through lines. Maintain good spine posture.

Breath of Life - Natural Breath Movement (Lom Haichai)
Fuel your body with life force by breathing deeply.

Mindfulness (Khwam Mi Sati)
If your mind starts to wander into the past or future, let those thoughts come and go and return to present moment awareness.

Positive Thinking (Kan Mong Lok Nai Ngae Di)
Remain positive through the tough times. Be patient. Have faith and confidence in yourself. Visualize the ideal posture.

Balance (Sama Dun)
Train everything equally, working on any imbalances if necessary. Use softness to balance and connect to the earth.

Relax (Kan Phon Khlai)
Only use what you need to use. Scan your body to feel for tension and if unsure tense and release.

All the essentials of Muay training are required as they complement each other. Explore yourself and do not limit yourself. Be satisfied and aim to do a little more.

Training in Daily Life

There are no limitations on when you can practise mindfulness, positive thinking, breathing, channelling and intensifying life force, balance, relaxation and cat stretches.

Health is Wealth

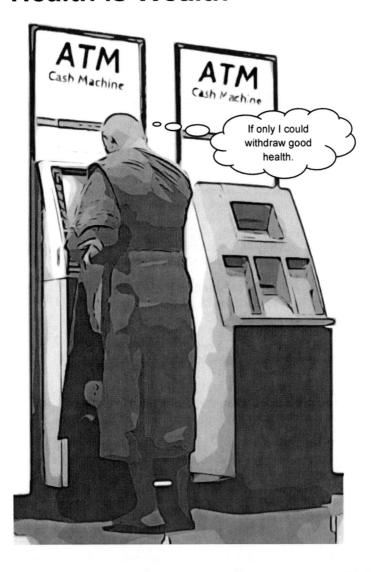

The reality of it is, you cannot buy good health and there is no quick fix.

Progression

The Muay warrior always aims to challenge themselves, they believe in continual change and development. Comfort zones and stagnation are not the way of Muay.

Training well at the edge (awareness zone) is essential to progress.

Challenge- Pick something you would like to gain or improve. Train on it every day or at least every other day. You will gain faith and confidence that your body will change and the results can be very rewarding.

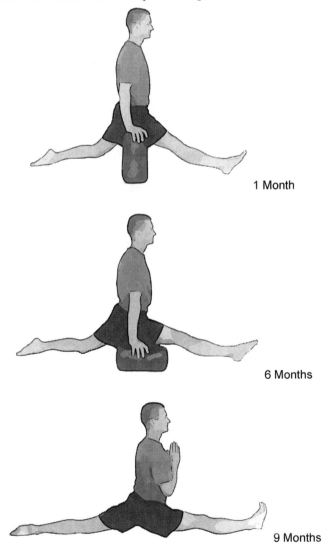

1 Month

6 Months

9 Months

Important Note- The body and mind will slowly adapt and progress with good habits, consistency, persistence and practice.

Aim to do a little more each session or at least once a week. It is normal for quick progression over the initial weeks. If progression slows down, remain positive and do not give up.

Consistency and persistence will change your mind and body, in the same way water carves its way through rock.

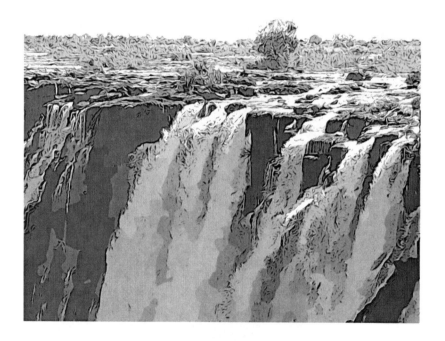

Warning- Start slowly and use your awareness to make sure what you practise is correct before you repeat it. It is about creating good habits, not bad ones.

Train, do not strain.

Remember, do not battle with yourself, use oneness and your energy wisely.

Nine Lethal and Easy to Learn Muay Strikes

The nine strikes have been included as an introduction to the self-defence techniques of Muay. They have been selected for being simple to use and very effective in self-defence.

There are techniques in Muay that are even more deadly than these that can take many months to master but you can master these nine strikes almost immediately, so you are able to defend yourself right from the very start of your training. Many lethal techniques in Muay were designed with a simple movement and so allowing soldiers to prepare for battle quickly. Many of these movements are practised in the Muay postures.

From these nine strikes you can advance in the thousands of other techniques.

If you fail with any of the strikes or even a combination of them, go for a bear hug. Remember though, the easiest way to defend yourself is to move out of the way.

Why Nine?

Gao meaning nine is an auspicious number for Thai people. It sounds the same as the Thai word *gaao* meaning to advance or progress forward.

Gao, when written in Thai, looks very much like the *unalom* symbol. *Unalom* is the mind's eye. It allows communication between the mind and body. It is the aura of power. A Muay Thai warrior always protects their *unalom* with their guard.

For these reasons, it is traditional for Muay students to give an offering of something to the value of nine to their teachers before they begin training.

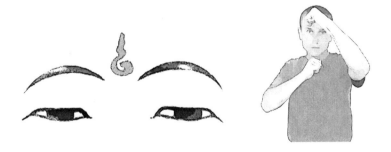

What if the Strikes Fail?

You need to be confident that the strikes will work but there is always a chance something could go wrong. If you get injured, worn out or overpowered and there is no opportunity to run away, you will need a backup plan. If all fails, a simple option is to go in for a bear hug. Once you have applied the bear hug it is important to keep moving. This will off-balance your opponent giving you more control and allowing you time to recover.

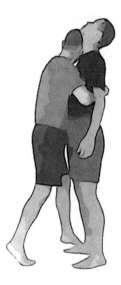

You can apply the bear hug over your opponent's arms giving them less chance to attack, or under their arms, where a tight squeeze will restrict their breathing. With either variation you must stay close to your opponent and if possible, aim to push your head under their chin. This will give you more protection and more control. For a good solid grip, grab your wrist.

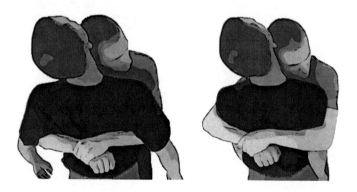

Combinations

Once you make a decision to attack, it is important not to stop moving until you have achieved peace or the chance to leave safely. If required you can use all the strikes in any combination.

All of the strikes can be followed with any another strike or repeated twice.

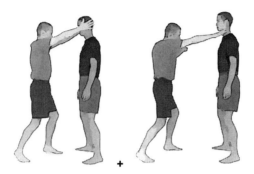

+

To advance, two or three strikes can be applied at the same time.

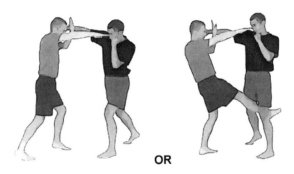

OR

Tips for All Strikes

- Maintain your feet in a triangular stance with your feet always shoulder width apart or wider.
- A small step forwards and turning the whole body as one will add extra power.
- Protect yourself and feel safe behind your guard.
- Create a loud noise when doing each technique to enhance power and confidence. It also serves to intimidate and distract your opponent.
- Strike with maximum speed and commitment.
- In a fight, commit yourself fully to the target area by being relaxed, balanced, positive and focused, striking through the target.
- All techniques have strengths and weaknesses. Become aware of this and use it to your advantage.
- Remember that confidence, positivity, patience and energy are all powerful weapons and allies of yours that will help you achieve peace.

All the strikes are extremely aggressive, wild looking and not pretty. It is important to stay in control of yourself, it may appear to others that you are not.

Warning for All Strikes

The strikes were designed for the Thai army for use on the battlefield. They are capable of causing serious or fatal injuries.

You and only you, the reader must be responsible for your own actions and safety when practising or using any of the techniques in this book. You must also adhere to and be aware of the law in regards to self-defence.

Be extra careful whilst practising during training and if possible avoid contact.

The Techniques

Sweep the Earth

Target: Knee joint.

How: Take a big step to the side of your opponent to avoid an attack and also to load up a low round kick. Swing your leg round striking with your shin. Pivot on the ball of your foot so that your whole body can turn as one.

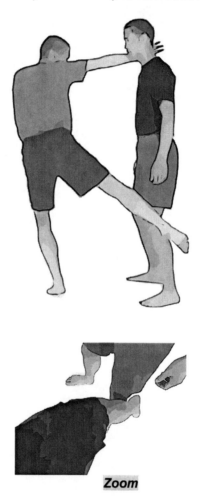

Zoom

Focus: Lean your body weight into the kick. It is a similar movement to kicking a ball as far as possible.

Interest: Also called Burst the Tyres because a fighter cannot fight without the use of his legs. A similar technique is called Senior Monk Sweeps the Grounds, where you respond to an opponent's high kick with a low round kick to their supporting leg.

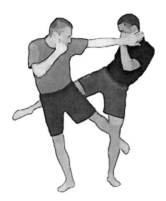

Variation: Can be used in combination with a defensive or attacking movement. By swinging your arm in the opposite direction, this can act as an extended guard to deflect attacks or to strike your opponent's head.

Variation: Another way to put your opponent's legs out of action is to push kick or side push kick their knee joint. More accuracy is required for this option.

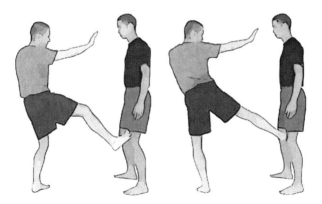

Split the Betel Nut

Target: Groin.

How: Raise your leg up to form a straight kick using your shin or foot as the weapon. Maintain a good guard and keep your leg straight with just a slight bend at the knee. Lean back slightly as you kick.

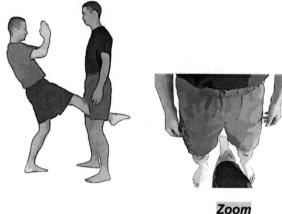

Zoom

Focus: To help commit yourself fully, intend to strike up through your opponent's groin and to their head.

Interest: The betel nut is an extremely hard to nut to crack! The swollen ripened fruit ranges from red to orange in colour. The picture shows a betel nut being sliced and prepared for chewing. It is a mental stimulant which, when chewed, stains the teeth, gums and lips a bright red colour.

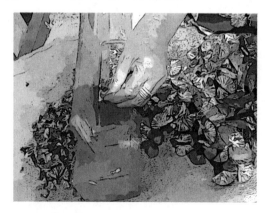

Variation: If you are at close range and you miss with your shin, you can strike with your knee instead.

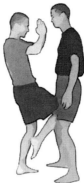

Variation: Swing one arm back for extra power.

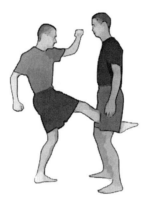

Variation: Can be used in combination with defensive movements.

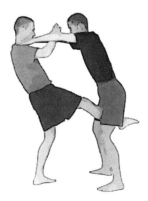

Charging Army

Target: Multiple parts of the body.

How: This strike can be as simple as swinging the arms across your body and as advanced as launching six strikes simultaneously. When using the basic arm swing, aim to strike with your outer wrist followed by your inner wrist of your other arm. Depending on your range, you can also strike with the outer edges of your hands or elbows. To complete the strike, you have to swing back round giving you a total of four strikes.

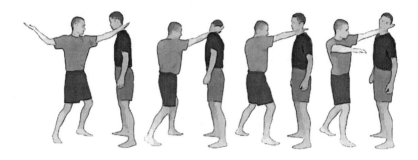

Focus: For speed and power maintain softness in the body.

Variation: The swing can also be used to deflect an opponent's attacking movements.

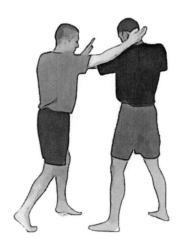

Variation: The advanced version includes launching a round kick at the same time, then landing forwards and repeating on the other side. If you are at a closer range you can use your knees and elbows to strike.

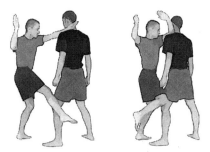

Interest: The movement originates from an attack pattern that was used by the Thai army to charge at the enemy. Weapons were also used which gave them extra range and making the strikes even more lethal.

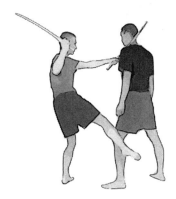

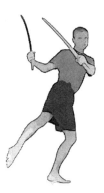

Repel the Tiger

Target: Neck.

How: Jab the inner edge of your index finger and thumb forwards, turning your whole body as one.

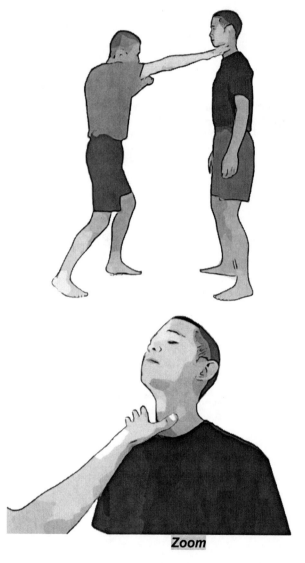

Zoom

Focus: Your finger and thumb need to be wide. Stay relaxed to increase speed.

Variation: Can be used in defence against a swing punch or straight punch by raising your elbow high at the same time as you strike, so that it blocks the incoming punch by making contact with your elbow.

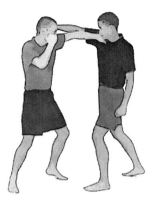

Variation: A similar technique is called Khmer Supports the Pillar which is a palm strike targeting the chin and neck. This leaves the opponent wide open for another strike. The Khmer was an ancient empire which included parts of Cambodia, Thailand, Laos and Vietnam.

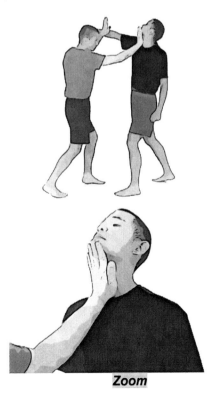

Zoom

Monkey Swings Revered Sword

Target: Ears.

How: Open your guard wide and then slam your palms together.

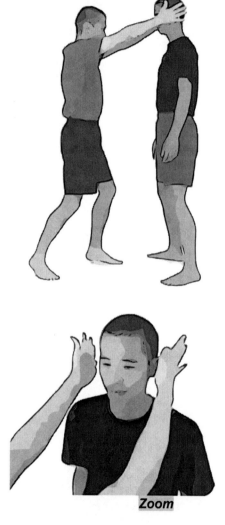

Zoom

Focus: Once you have applied this strike you must back away fast or apply your next move.

Interest: The green monkey king in this technique is called Ongkot. He is Hanuman's cousin and the son of the green monkey king Pali. Ongkot is a noble warrior and friend of King Rama. He is rewarded a great title for being successful in the battle of Lanka.

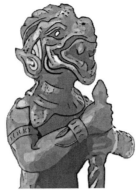

Variation: If someone goes to grab you low, it will give you the perfect opportunity to apply this strike.

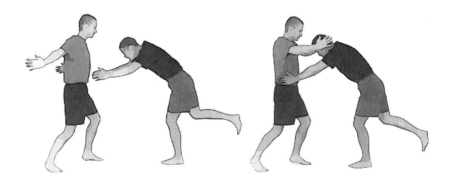

Variation: Another option is to strike with your fists or inner wrists. Other targets are your opponent's temples or neck.

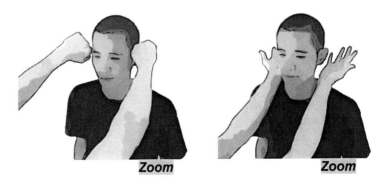

Zoom   Zoom

Prepare for Battle

Target: Head.

How: Grab your opponent's head, then simultaneously pull down and strike with a round elbow. The elbow travels up and down.

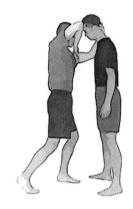

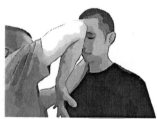

Zoom

Focus: The more you can deliver the round elbow strike vertically downwards, the more powerful it will be. Use equal amount of energy inwards with both arms.

Interest: All nine strikes are designed for simplicity so they are quick to learn. The advantage of this was so that the Thai military could prepare themselves for battle quickly and effectively.

Force the Elephant Down

Target: Head.

How: Grab your opponent's neck. For the best grip hold on to your wrist. Force your opponent's head down whilst at the same time thrusting you knee straight up.

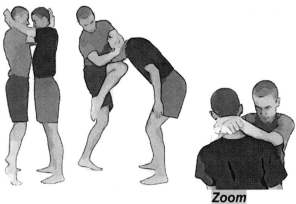

Zoom

Focus: To help commit yourself fully it is good to be aware that if the movement continues without impact, your arms will travel down to the same side of your body that you knee with.

Interest: The name of the technique comes from the Ramakien story when Hanuman (Monkey God) battles with Erawan (elephant). Eventually, Hanuman breaks Erawan's neck. Erawan has thirty-three heads but is often depicted with only three and was used by Indra (God of War) as a means of transport.

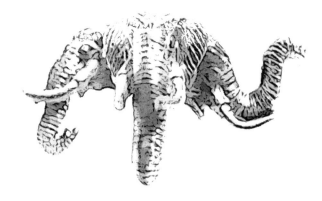

Playful Singing of the Mynah Bird

Target: Multiple parts of the body.

How: Use repetitive chopping like movements with the inner edge of the wrist or hand. The chops can also include strikes aiming at your opponent's attacking strikes.

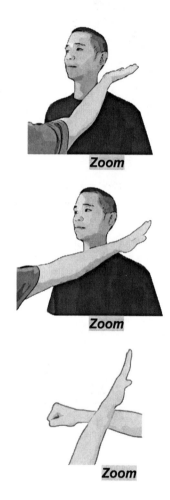

Zoom

Zoom

Zoom

Focus: Must be fast and continuous.

Interest: This technique involves repeated defensive or attacking strikes, all using chops with the inner wrist. Chopping with the inner wrist bone delivers a nasty strike and is a lot safer than a punch. With a punch it is easy to break bones in the hand.

This style mimics the nature of the Mynah bird, which is known in Thailand for making annoying repetitive noises. The bird appears to play a game with you by copying what you say repetitively.

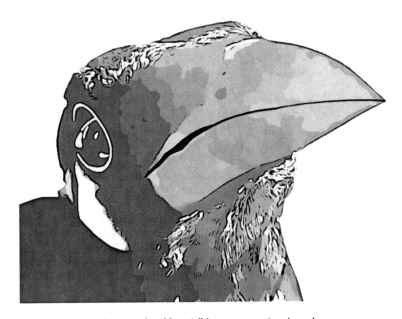

The technique can be practised by striking your partner's palms.

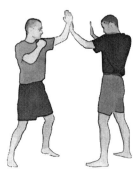

A single strike to the neck is called Cutting Off the Fish Head. Close your fist and it becomes a strike called Elephant Thrashes its Trunk. A similar technique is called the Burmese Axe Dance, again with the fist closed, using the inner wrist as an extension of the weapon.

Tiger Claws

Target: Eyes.

How: Thrust your fingers forward in the shape of tigers claws.

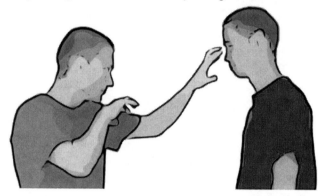

Focus: Using both hands to claw will increase your chance of a successful strike.

Interest: It is believed that there was an ancient technique used called Tiger Sharpens its Claws. This was an attack pattern of rotating the guard so that the bound fists would roll down continually over the opponents face or body. The knots on the knuckles of the fists would cause tiger like scratches. The fists were bound in wraps made with horse hide or hemp and sprayed with water, forming a nasty weapon as well as giving firm protection.

It is said that you should keep your knowledge and practice of Muay a secret, in the same way a tiger's claws are hidden when not needed. Bragging and telling others is not the way of the Muay masters.

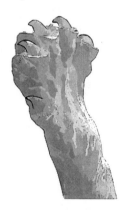

Variation: The hands can be straight or in the shape of a bird's beak.

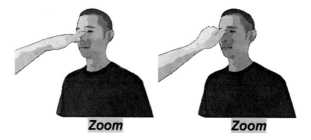

Variation: The double eye poke technique is called Rahu Swallows Moon. You can also use your thumbs.

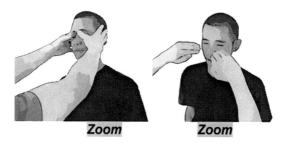

Interest: In ancient times Thai people believed that the moon deity, Rahu caused the eclipses of the sun. Rahu is half ogre, half human.

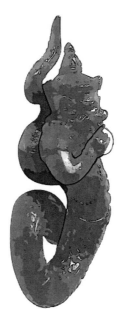

Muaythai Institute

Recognized by the
World Muaythai Council
Ministry of Education

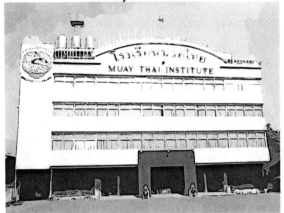

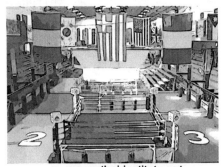

www.muaythai-institute.net
E-mail: muaythai911@hotmail.com
Address: 323 Prahonyothin 119 Pahonyothin Road Prachatipat Thayaburee
Prathumthanee Rangsit Thailand 12130

Luktupfah Muaythai Camp and Institute of Thai Martial Arts

Recognized by the
Kru Muaythai Association
The Conservation Institution of Muay Thai Chaiya
World Muay Boran Federation and World Muaythai Federation

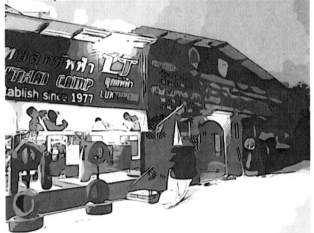

www.luktupfah-muaythai.com
E-mail: luktupfah_muaythai@hotmail.com
Address: 5 Onnut 65 Soi 8 Pravet Bangkok Thailand

About the Author

Lee has been training in martial arts since the age of 7 and gained a black belt when he was 12 years old.

His professional Muay Thai fight led to television appearances in four Thai programmes and two advertisements.

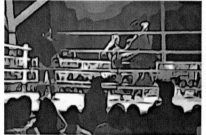 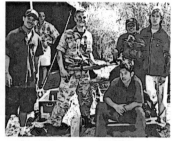

After fighting professionally, Lee trained to become a teacher and received certification from the Ministry of Education and the World Muaythai Council at the Muaythai Institute in Thailand.

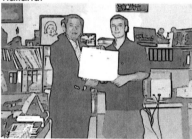

Lee has studied and practised Muay Thai and Muay Boran intensively at many gyms/camps in Thailand.

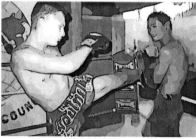

He has taught Muay in Thailand and the UK since 2000.

In 2006, Lee qualified as a Yoga teacher in India. He has also trained with masters from around the world in various traditional martial arts, including Kalarippayattu in India, Kung Fu in China and Capoeira in Brazil.

มวย

CPSIA information can be obtained at www.ICGtesting.com
Printed in the USA
LVOW12s1503070615

441507LV00001B/266/P